Bhakti Flow Yoga

Bhakti Flow YOGA

A Training Guide
for Practice and Life

RUSTY WELLS

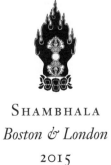

SHAMBHALA
Boston & London
2015

Shambhala Publications, Inc.
Horticultural Hall
300 Massachusetts Avenue
Boston, Massachusetts 02115
www.shambhala.com

9 8 7 6 5 4 3 2 1

FIRST EDITION
Printed in the United States of America

⊗ This edition is printed on acid-free paper that meets the
American National Standards Institute z39.48 Standard.
♲ This book is printed on 30% postconsumer recycled paper.
For more information please visit www.shambhala.com.

Distributed in the United States by Penguin Random House LLC
and in Canada by Random House of Canada Ltd

Photos by Thayer Allyson Gowdy
Designed by Steve Dyer

Library of Congress Cataloging-in-Publication Data

Wells, Rusty, author.
Bhakti flow yoga: a training guide for practice and life / Rusty Wells.
—First edition.
pages   cm
ISBN 978-1-61180-239-9 (paperback: alk. paper)
1. Yoga. 2. Yoga, Bhakti. I. Title.
RA781.67W45 2015
613.7′046—dc23
2014045304

INVOCATION

May we know God's love,
the God of each our own unique understanding,
in every heartbeat and breath.

In every thought and the spaces between our thoughts.
In every whisper, utterance, and song.
In every waking moment and deep within our sleep.

In our movement and in our stillness.
As we eat and drink.
As we make peace and as we make love.

May we take refuge here, in the heart of the Beloved.
And may we always bow humbly forward with gratitude for
*   having this love.*
I pray that this book, in some small or some magnificent way,
leads you a little closer toward the God of your own sweet
*   understanding.*
I offer this work to my teachers. I am always at your feet.

RUSTY (GOPA)

Contents

Bhakti Flow Yoga

Welcome

We shall not cease from exploration
And the end of all our exploring
Will be to arrive where we started
And know the place for the first time.

—T. S. ELIOT, *Four Quartets*

THIS BOOK is designed to share what I have learned so far through my personal yoga path and spiritual quest. I am excited to introduce this practice to anyone who is interested in learning more about yoga. My experience with the practice has brought me great awareness, purpose, connectedness, and delight. Still, I do not pretend to know everything there is to know about the art and science of yoga. In fact, I consider myself quite the beginner. But, to date, I have certainly enjoyed a unique adventure, one that seems to have resonated with many other like-hearted beings in classes I lead in San Francisco and in programs and training sessions I conduct around the world.

After nearly two decades of being a yoga practitioner, my own practice still invariably begins with starting over each and every day. This may seem counterintuitive. After all, yoga is an age-old system of well-being that consists of practicing and repeating many of the same techniques again and again. As our practice develops through days and months and years, we see our physical asana improving; our lungs expanding; our minds evolving; and our ability to feel compassion, patience, and virtue increasing. Yet in my practice, and from what I have witnessed while leading students all these years, the true key to an "advanced state of practice" seems to be the constant willingness to begin again.

The practice of yoga is the ultimate art of paying attention to the *now*. How precious it is when we can truly be present in every moment with the most loving and compassionate attitude toward ourselves and others. This very attitude is how beginners often enter the practice. They have no choice; they don't know what else to expect. A beginner's inherent present-mind awareness, the raw tendency to be absolutely in the body and in the moment without expectation, is at the very heart of the Bhakti Flow experience. When we are so in awe of the wonder of this moment that we can't help but savor its freshness, its newness, even its bittersweet brevity, that's when we are most alive. When we retain the beginner's willingness for adventure and the ability to feel our experience viscerally in every moment, the practice stays fresh and becomes so incredibly vast.

After all, we should never forget that every day is a gift waiting to unfold, to be unwrapped. It's impossible for one day to be the same as another. In fact, the only thing I know for certain is real is *this very moment*. The memory of yesterday is merely that, a memory. The hopes of tomorrow are not guaranteed. But this moment, with everything that I can ponder and see and taste and feel and touch and embrace and speak to and listen to and even smell, is real. I pay great respect to every experience that has brought me to this present moment, knowing that my past—no matter what my feelings of attachment, avoidance, or even indifference toward parts of it may be—has happened for some great purpose that is unfolding to me even in this very moment.

Every day, I begin my asana practice anew. I think, *I have never stood in this Mountain Pose before. I have never felt this Downward-Facing Dog Pose before. I have never breathed this one breath. My dedication, my very intention behind the practice, has never mattered more than now. I remain hopeful, but I also let go of any expectations about where I think I should be in this pose or where I have been before in this pose or where I want to go in this pose later. I demand nothing from this pose.* I choose to listen to my body and breath and heart and let that guide me. As a beginner, I allow myself the opportunity to inquire and open. But I always do my work so that I may establish strength and balance in my foundation and use all the tools I've been given. In this way, I set the stage for truly being present in the mystical wonder of living in this moment and in life itself.

Here in the West, there is often an emphasis on the physical branch of practice, namely Hatha Yoga. Because of this, many people think that yoga is primarily about physical contortionism. In reality, it is more about contortions of the mind: the twisting and churning, the considering and reconsidering, the allowing and accepting, the appetite and aptitude, the patience and perseverance. These are the elements of yoga that ultimately bring health and healing to our bodies, minds, and hearts. This true flexibility, that of mind and spirit, is what helps heal our personal relationships, our communities, and the world. One of the greatest yogis, Mahatma Gandhi, primarily taught and lived by the very first root of the first limb of the Yoga Sutras: *ahimsa*, or nonharming. Gandhi's devotion to pacifism and reform through example meant that he lived his entire life by this one yogic principle and in so doing created a complete practice for himself and many others. We didn't need to see him twist his body into a pretzel to recognize how he changed the world with his yoga practice.

I invite you to sit back and enjoy this book but then get ready to take these practices to your yoga mat and out into your everyday life. The greatest changes in history have always begun with the efforts of one devoted individual. Remember that today is a gift you will never get back; part of this gift is the option to begin again. For those who have ever felt off-center or alone, I invite you to take comfort here.

Before we begin—a note on the G word. The word we use to refer to the divine can be highly charged for some people. This is really the "God" of your own unique and highly personal understanding. I use the word *God* for lack of any better word to describe the wonder that is this beautiful truth. If this word does not resonate with you, please feel free to substitute any word you prefer: Beloved, Mother Earth, friend, nature. Anything that is meaningful to you is perfect.

PART ONE

Foundations and Philosophy

CHAPTER 1

Bhakti Flow Yoga

ONE OF MY FAVORITE IMAGES in all of yoga has nothing to do with a yoga pose. I am thinking of the beautiful image of Krishna and Radha in a deep embrace. This image depicts an eternal exchange of love. There is something so connected between the lover and the beloved that the two become one in a manner that transcends basic human materialism. This is *krishna-bhakti*, the love of Krishna. I see in this embrace an empowerment and equality that is quite special.

If you can recall a moment when you felt truly loved and felt that you mattered more than you had ever realized, you may begin to understand what this embrace is about. In that awareness of pure love, we set aside every doubt and insecurity and, for perhaps one splendid moment, allow ourselves to be beautiful and worthy. To me, it is as if the divine places a gentle kiss upon our brow, reminding us that we are here for a purpose and that we matter more than we may understand.

This image has greatly influenced my yoga practice and the creation of Bhakti Flow Yoga, which is my own heart-child—a combination of Bhakti Yoga and Vinyasa Flow. I wanted to find a way to achieve harmony and grace in a contemporary urban context. *Bhakti* refers to the yoga of love and devotion, while *flow* refers to the seamless connection between the breath and the movements of the body. This is also called *vinyasa*. Students experience a dancelike quality in the practice, involving a creative and continuous deepening of the yoga poses in an effort to attain present-time awareness. It is also an energetic response, during which you have the opportunity to open up and observe. Whether you are in a pose that you love or one that you may not like quite as much, flow is about bringing all that stuff to the surface so you can be with it as it is.

By definition, yet without reference to religious conventionalism or dogma, Bhakti Flow Yoga is a dance-filled prayer, a movement that brings each of us closer to the God of our own understanding. This point is very important. How you personally connect with the divine is what matters. Some people have a deity, others have elements of nature, and some see the light of the divine in the eyes of their partner or children. Native Americans have eloquently called this "acknowledging the Wonder." For me, this Wonder is the invisible hand that guides me to all things great and good. If you follow a specific religion, you are invited to place the devotion as you would in your religion. If you are not religious, you are invited to enjoy the same benefits of this nonsectarian spiritual practice without the slightest orthodoxy.

I pay homage to the many systems of Hatha Yoga that offer specific, sometimes even strict, sequences of yoga poses. I've been inspired by many of these systems over the years, but ultimately I have felt hampered by certain rigidities and systematic structures that can turn into something that feels almost like religion. These systems of Hatha Yoga work wonderfully for a lot of people. But for me and others like me, there are alternative paths; the path that nurtures my complete being is Bhakti Flow. This yoga is liberated and powerful. It allows creative self-expression to blossom unapologetically and unabashedly. Ultimately, it helps us find our place in this world so we can move through life with great kindness and no regret.

Some systems of yoga do not address natural human emotions, yet emotions are an integral part of who we are individually and collectively. In Bhakti Flow, we look at the whole—the mind, the body, and the heart—and do our best to integrate this into the complete experience. It is from here that we discover a sacred and personal understanding of who we really are. The flow invites us to keep moving compassionately through our observations, becoming more aware of our avoidances and our attachments. This empowers us to make better choices in our lives, choices that will inevitably enrich us, our families, and our communities.

The awakening of compassion, kindness, and gratitude is integral to the experience. The emphasis is on letting go of narrow, selfish motives and learning to live fully in the present. Practitioners progress not simply through the attainment of asana, but through the belief that they can improve their own lives—as well as the lives of others—by being gentler, kinder, and more caring. There is an emphasis on *ahimsa* (nonharming) while considering the happiness and well-being of others. In a sense, the practice itself is akin to a supportive and liberating universal hug.

In Bhakti Flow Yoga classes, my goal is to create and foster a space that brings the openness of the embrace between Krishna and Radha: a big hug that is all-inclusive, clear-eyed, and uplifting for everyone. An embrace that empowers and emboldens and provides a safe refuge. As we prepare for class, we keep this in mind. The lighting, the sound, the smell—and even more important, how our community is greeted—play an integral part in this welcoming embrace. From their first step inside to the moment they leave our care, all guests are treated with equal loving-kindness.

The embrace of Krishna and Radha reminds me that no matter what this life hands me in all its many glories and inevitable defeats, I am never really alone. I am always held in a supreme embrace by a creator who has given me breath and life for a purpose that is all my own to understand. All I need to do is open my eyes and my heart.

To me, the practice of Bhakti Flow is about discovering ways to reconnect to that divine spark in all my relationships. Krishna makes it clear that his presence is in all beings. We are welcome to call him anything we like. We can see him in any manner we wish. And my favorite part is that there is an equal amount of his love and divinity in all beings. No one has any more than anyone else. And no one has any less than anyone else. We are equal. It's as simple as that. If we assume someone else has more of the divine presence in them, we lessen our own purpose in this life and hence dim a light that should really only shine brighter. I like to recommend to students that if they meet someone who claims to have more than they do, they consider smiling at the person and running away.

My Path to Yoga

I practice, teach, and live Bhakti Yoga, the yoga of love and devotion. I was first introduced to this practice in 1990, before I tried any Hatha Yoga at all. This compassionate practice follows Lord Krishna's teachings, which are at the heart of the Bhagavad Gita: *Bhaktya mam abhijanati* (18:11), which means "I can only be known by devotional service." These teachings have also shown me the importance of other aspects of *bhakti* such as selfless service (*seva*) and chanting in a group (*kirtan*) or softly to oneself (*japa*).

I was already in love with Bhakti Yoga when some of my pals, who were yoga teachers, started talking to me about Hatha Yoga. Or, more accurately, nagging me (for a long time!) to just *try* this other form of yoga. I would roll my eyes at them. But finally, due to their insistence, I went—kicking and screaming. To my great surprise, I immediately found it to be a profound experience; I felt as though I were in a noncompetitive environment for the first time in my life. It felt safe, like a really creative place to go and release something. Because of this, I kept going back, and I stayed in the practice with great humility and appreciation. To this day, when I thank my teachers, I always think of those first teacher friends who insisted I try it. They fed me in countless ways, and I also believe they are somewhat tickled (and maybe a little perplexed) at what they started.

I've now been teaching in the San Francisco Bay Area since 1998, and I also teach this method of yoga internationally. I enjoy fusing together the many wonderful influences I've had over the years from diverse and inspiring teachers. These teachers include not just yoga instructors, but everyone who has ever demonstrated patience and exquisite kindness, including every parent who somehow "keeps it all together." Their eclectic methods inspire my teaching and continue to deepen the experiences of my own personal practice, and I am eternally grateful to them.

The Practice of Bhakti Flow Yoga

The public classes I lead incorporate techniques that bring us to a state of present-time awareness, breathing space into our lives where we can find compassion, love, and great gratitude. If you were to join us for a class or workshop in San Francisco—or elsewhere in the world—here is roughly what you would experience.

At the start of the class, I ask folks to meet someone they do not know. There is an immediate electric energy in the room when this happens, a sense of excitement and connection. It takes a few minutes for what I call "fellowship"—when people introduce themselves—and then the subsequent settling back into their own spaces. This time sets the tone for the practice and leads into the dedication, in which everyone has the opportunity to dedicate their practice to whatever intention they choose. If people have devotion in their lives, they know where to focus. If not, we simply encourage them to send that intention to someone they may care for dearly or even someone they simply want to see happier, healthier, and free from harm.

Most of the classes are celebratory, so excitement tends to fill the air from the start. As we move through the practice, the tone moves to one of focused work and then graduates into a more playful aspect of work. From here, we wind down to a moment of peaceful surrender, only to be reawakened with loving care back to the excitement from which the experience was first born.

We keep the room warm but not stifling. The heat is on throughout, but we also keep windows ajar and ceiling fans on to keep fresh air moving and the humidity level within reason. Many of the classes use music to deepen the experience. I personally play just about every form of music in my classes, and I believe that most music has the potential to bring healing or awareness. I encourage newer teachers to build trust with the student community first and try not to freak them out too early. The music is intended to be complementary to the experience without overshadowing it.

The poses we practice are wide-ranging, an array of traditional poses often interspersed with those that are unique and innovative. We offer variations for those exploring different phases in their practice, as well as modifications for those new to the experience or who might need to practice in a more conservative manner. We teach and practice *ahimsa*. Knowing that many students come in with a set attitude to work superhard, we do our best to counter that by reminding them how important it is to find a healthy and safe balance in the practice. This mental adjustment strips away any competitive insistence, either with others or with themselves.

My assistants and I wander the room, offering hands-on and verbal adjustments. But we make it clear that students should feel comfortable declining this offer, either verbally or by placing one of our "No thanks, No touch" chips in clear view on their mat.

At its heart, what makes something a Bhakti Flow class is the purpose behind the action. This is why each class begins and ends with dedication. It is a very personal and profound moment, as students place that intention where they most want it. Throughout the practice, we ask students to remember their intention and connect what they are doing in the moment to that intention. One mission statement of Bhakti Flow is that it's not about simply bringing you a healthier body and peace of mind. These are just by-products of the practice. The aim of the practice is about experiencing real connection and enlightenment (oneness), which we refer to as *samadhi*. The gifts of this mystical journey just so happen to include a radiant body and a joyful existence. This practice is also about finding devotion in our lives, a devotion defined only by our own unique understanding. We simply hold the space for creative self-expression to emerge.

Bhakti Flow is a place to begin again, yet it is not confined to the yoga mat. It is a way of life. It is a way of interacting. It is about how we look at all of our personal relationships: with family, with friends, with those who challenge us, even with those we don't know. More broadly, this also includes our relationships to our past, our work, our environment, our bodies, our food, our money, and even our long-held faith systems. Through the practice, we look at all of these things with minds that are open, hearts that are willing, and eyes that are clear. As we look at them, these things may or may not come to hold the same meaning they once did.

So while you may come to the mat to get stretchy and gorgeous—and that's okay!—remember that these are just side benefits of the practice. When we become more flexible, we become more reasonable. When we become stronger, we can find the fortitude to stand up against injustice. When we find balance on the mat, balance seems to find us off the mat as well.

CHAPTER 2

Origins and History

I am the beginning and the end,
origin and dissolution,
refuge, home, true lover, womb and imperishable seed.

— BHAGAVAD GITA (9:18)

BHAKTI YOGA AND VINYASA FLOW, the two elements that fuse together to create Bhakti Flow Yoga, both have rich and colorful his-
tories. In fact, all of yoga has a rich and colorful history! While historical
knowledge is not necessary to benefit from or enjoy this (or any) style
of yoga, an understanding of what came before can make the experience
even deeper.

India, the birthplace of yoga, is an ancient land where spiritual associations run deep. Through millennia, its people have pondered the purpose
of life and wondered about the highest possibilities of the human mind.
Why are we born human? Where have we come from? What is life all
about? Where do we go from here? What happens after we die? Yoga,
in its purest form, offers a path to ultimate realization. It emphasizes action and practice: liberation comes through one's own work. There is no
other way. The roots of this ancient practice reach far and wide, allowing a myriad of seekers to experience for themselves the most joyous life
possible.

Yoga itself seems to have begun between 3000 and 1900 B.C.E. The
exact date isn't important; what *is* important is that yoga speaks to the
development of consciousness, and through that development comes im-
provement of the human condition. Imagine how things could change for
the better if more people took to practicing yoga correctly and sincerely.
Their lives would improve, as would the lives of those with whom they

interact. As we begin to take care of ourselves, we lift ourselves up. When we lift ourselves, we can then lift up our families and friends, our work-places, and our communities.

For ease of understanding, the development of yoga is classified into four periods: Vedic; Preclassical; Classical; and Postclassical, which leads into modern yoga. Through the ages, yoga has been practiced and under-stood in different ways. In fact, with its emphasis on practice and personal experience, yoga actually encourages each practitioner to find his or her own path. This is why so many different kinds of yoga are available today, and this dogma-free approach is part of what has made yoga such a bless-ing to so many people.

The Vedic period takes its name from the Vedas. These ancient Brah-manical scriptures, presented as hymns, contain the earliest known yogic teachings, recounting personal experiences with divine truth.

From what we know, Vedic yoga evolved around rituals that were seen as a way to transcend material limitations and connect with the spirit. It was crucial for the yogi to concentrate deeply for long periods of time. Such deep concentration is one of the essential practices of yoga; it is the tool that enables us to explore the innermost recesses of the mind. In the classes I offer, I often remind people that the practice is not about the body. It's not about the heat, the sweat, or even the music. It's about what the mind is doing in each moment. Is it clinging to something? Is it running away? Do we even know what we are thinking? Being aware of our thoughts and shifting them, if need be, is what matters.

The Upanishads are the primary texts of Preclassical yoga. They num-ber more than two hundred and are akin to snapshots of vivid spiritual insights; they do not offer clear explanations or a systematic flow of con-cepts, but rather the yogis' impressions of divine truth or ultimate reality. It's interesting to note that this divine truth is presented in different ways. This is possibly the result of seers experiencing truth from various levels of spiritual awareness or perhaps just describing truth in their own specific ways. Whatever the reason for the differing descriptions, the important point is the central message of the Upanishads: the underlying concepts of *brahman* (ultimate reality); *atman* (each individual's divine consciousness); dharma (the law of nature); karma (the law of cause and effect); *samsara* (the cycle of birth and death); and *moksha* (liberation). These are each fundamental yogic concepts, but none of them are independent from the others because everything in the universe is interconnected. We are all parts of a whole.

The first written mention of Bhakti Yoga appears during this period in the Bhagavad Gita, which probably dates to around 500 B.C.E. The Gita, one section of one of the Upanishads, imparts knowledge about *brahma-vidya* (the supreme science of yoga) in the form of a dialogue between the god Krishna and the warrior Arjuna. This dialogue can be understood as the struggle to rise above craving, ignorance, and aversion to realize the highest truth. It is symbolic of the struggle that ensues within each of us, showing a way to confront the forces of evil within and without and to overcome these forces through positive action. The Gita urges us to self-less action with the best of motives and without ego.

In moments of deep meditation, yogis have discovered that the Self does not differ from person to person; rather, it is the same in all creatures. In the Bhagavad Gita, Krishna says to Arjuna,

> I am the true Self in the heart of every creature, Arjuna,
> And the beginning, middle and end of their existence.
>
> — BHAGAVAD GITA (10:20)

A fully enlightened person is capable of unconditional compassion because such a being is free from craving, aversion, and ignorance:

> [When a person]
> . . . responds to the joys and sorrows of others as if they were
>   his own,
> He has attained the highest state of spiritual union.
>
> — BHAGAVAD GITA (6:32)

In the Gita, Krishna explains four approaches: Karma Yoga, Jnana Yoga, Raja Yoga, and Bhakti Yoga. The goal of all four paths is the same—direct experience of divine consciousness or divine Self, which can be achieved only when the mind is completely free and totally pure. Yet each approach emphasizes a different method.

The Karma yogi takes the path of selfless action. Development on this path comes through renunciation of selfish attachment to the outcome of any action; the concept is to work single-mindedly and altruistically, without thought of personal gain or gratification of ego. The true Karma yogi strives to rise above ego and to work for the divine, for the good of all beings. This is an excellent path for those who live in the material world, as the practitioner's daily work becomes the path.

Jnana Yoga is the yoga of knowledge acquired through developing the power of discernment. The Jnana yogi aspires to employ willpower and discriminating wisdom to view everything from a position of detachment.

Raja Yoga is the science of meditation, of disciplining the mind through concentration and right awareness of the senses. Hatha Yoga comes from Raja Yoga, and Vinyasa Yoga sits under the umbrella of Hatha Yoga.

Bhakti Yoga is the yoga that brings me home, the inspiration for the practice I call Bhakti Flow Yoga. The Bhakti yogi aspires to identify with the divine through complete devotion, by loving God totally and unconditionally. Love is a powerful motivator and can inspire practitioners to realize their divine potential. When we love selflessly, it is a divine love, the love that is referred to as *bhakti* in the Bhagavad Gita. We see divinity in every aspect of the universe and can do no harm to ourselves or others.

Traditional Bhakti practices include the repetition of a mantra, either silently to oneself or aloud in a group; the drawing of inspiration from sacred texts and meditation; and a lifestyle that has much to do with self-less acts of service as well as with a diet based on nonharming and good health. In Bhakti Flow Yoga, we sing together and sweat together and focus on how our practice can bring goodness and healing into the lives of others. We even discuss how our diet can be in harmony with taking care of ourselves and the planet. The universal connection between all of these practices is integral to the Bhakti Flow experience. But remember: there is no need for dogma in any of this. If you are exploring this practice, I encourage you to study some of the traditions but eventually feel free to allow your own creative self-expression to help make it fit into your life.

The Divine in Bhakti Flow Yoga

The stories and fables of Hinduism bring a colorful and inspiring perspective to my practice both on and off the mat. These attempts to describe the indescribable offer me a helpful connection to how I offer my intentions, move through yoga poses, or navigate my way through everyday life. Trying to explain the inexplicable can be poetic, profound, and sometimes intentionally absurd. In the Hindu tradition, stories of the gods abound, offering a concept of God from a human perspective. Through stories, we can develop an understanding of the qualities that each Hindu deity represents, fostering a desire to connect with Divinity and imbibe these attributes through awareness and compassion. Tales that describe the accomplishments and virtues of the gods also inspire us to connect to the Divinity within, thus setting us on the path to full realization of God.

A stranger to Hindu philosophy might wonder at the concept of a pantheon of gods. However, this pantheon actually represents the various aspects of the *one* God, not a host of different deities. Hinduism—in its deep understanding of human nature, its compassion, and its flexibility—gives seekers the freedom to approach God through whichever aspect they find most familiar and inspiring. There are as many different forms as there are worshippers.

Scriptural stories do not just highlight the different aspects of God; they also demonstrate and honor the relationship between devotees and the divine. Many Hindu narratives exemplify the spiritual and sacrosanct love that flows between God and follower—that still moment when time ceases to exist, the sounds of the world fade away, and God stands before us with hands outstretched, offering blissful reunion. This is the path of *bhakti*. It is belonging to, being a part of, sharing in, and worshipping God. This all-embracing and complete awareness of God is reflected in the traditional Hindu greeting of *namaste*. Pressing your palms together in a praying gesture with head bowed and saying "*Namaste*" is not just a salutation; it is an active recognition of that divine spark of God that all living creatures carry within them.

The message at the heart of Bhakti stories is that the strength and sincerity of our devotion is what matters, that God will hear the devotee and respond with love. The true Bhakti practitioner views the material world with detachment, remaining secure in God's love. Residing in the heart of the believer, God—or the divine light—erases ignorance and shines through, emanating understanding and compassion. This path of Bhakti Yoga can lead us to the heart of the Beloved and the grace of God.

For me, there is also something fascinating about the connection between the stories of deities (God's different personalities) and certain yoga poses. When I think of Hanuman—a devotee of Rama and the epitome of devotion and service—and his great leaps of faith and courage, my splits become invigorated and much more hopeful. And when I am in Goddess Pose (Utkata Konasana), I can't help but consider my relationship and connection to the earth. As my hips sink toward the floor, I am not just taking the pose itself; I am assuming the role of caretaker for our earth. These thoughts guide me into the dynamic possibilities of every unique experience on the mat.

The Preclassical period also saw the establishment of a number of yoga schools, each of which developed various techniques of contemplation to enable yogis to transcend material reality and experience the ultimate truth. It was during this period that Gautama Buddha practiced yoga and attained enlightenment. The approach he followed and taught is known as the Noble Eightfold Path. The Buddha's unique and priceless contribution to yoga is the concept of *prajna* (wisdom). It is only through the development of *prajna* (or *panna* in Pali) that we can purify our minds.

The Noble Eightfold Path consists of the following precepts: right speech, right action, right livelihood, right effort, right awareness, right concentration, right thought, and right understanding. Having walked the path himself and achieved enlightenment, the Buddha knew each step, each obstacle, and every possible diversion. He also emphasized that it is up to the seeker to undertake this journey. The path taught by the Bhagavad Gita and the Buddha is not one of extreme indulgence or abstinence; it is the path of moderation, or the Middle Way.

The Buddha had a simple explanation for his approach:

> Abstain from all unwholesome deeds,
> Perform wholesome ones,
> Purify your mind.
>
> — DHAMMAPADA, XIV 5 (183)

Imagine if everyone the world over followed this simple prescription. The entire world would shift.

Foundations of Vinyasa Flow: Classical, Postclassical,
and Modern Yoga

The defining work of the Classical period is Patanjali's Yoga Sutras, which teach Raja Yoga, the eightfold approach to yoga. Composed in the second century C.E., this esoteric Sanskrit text contains around 195 brief lessons that have been the subject of much study and analysis through the ages. They outline a route to self-realization through meditation. Many serious students and practitioners of yoga refer to these sutras as the essential yogic text.

The instruction contained within the Yoga Sutras is generally known as Ashtanga Yoga, the eightfold path, because of its eight limbs, or principles: *yamas* (moral codes of conduct); *niyamas* (development of tolerance and purity); *asanas* (physical exercises and postures); *pranayama* (methods of breath control); *pratyahara* (preparation for meditation); *dharana* (method of concentration); *dhyana* (meditation); and *samadhi* (total concentration), which is the deepest stage of meditation. In Bhakti Flow Yoga, these eight limbs provide tools on which we regularly rely, although we take them in no particular order. And each of these tools is open to interpretation by the individual practitioner.

Yamas are guidelines that are meant to help us interact with the outside world and relate to others. They are not commandments but recommendations. Here is a list of the *yamas*:

1. *Ahimsa*, the principle of nonharming. Both the *yamas* and *niyamas* are rooted in *ahimsa*. The reality is that the very nature of life has harm, but by recognizing where this exists—and doing our best to create less harm in life—we begin to develop the quality of *ahimsa*. Kindness is central to growing in yoga. Every part of the practice has a foundation in *ahimsa* and kindness.
2. *Satya* refers to truthfulness in speech, thoughts, and actions.
3. *Asteya* essentially means nonstealing, noncoveting, and not being jealous.
4. *Brahmacharya* can be translated as "to act in the way of God." It implies exemplary conduct in all relationships, including our sexual associations. *Brahmacharya* is not about repression; it's about being able to recognize passion for what it is and develop a neutral response to it. It involves the wise use of energy and the control of sensual cravings.
5. *Aparigraha* means nonattachment. Developing a sense of nonattachment to possessions and people makes us happier and allows us to foster balanced and meaningful relationships.

Niyamas are guidelines meant to help us develop the internal discipline that is integral to spiritual growth. Regulating ourselves better enables us to maintain a positive environment in which to grow. The *niyamas* are as follows:

1. *Saucha* refers to purity and cleanliness of body, mind, and spirit.
2. *Santosha* (contentment) asks us to accept what is and make the best of everything. Living a life of gratitude is the source of joy and contentment. The key to happiness is in the mind.
3. *Tapas* has different meanings. It can mean "to heat" or "austerity." Some spiritual practices are known to generate heat in the body, which is indicative of development on the path. Spiritual austerity is empowering, and *tapas* also refers to this power. We can begin on this path by being disciplined and sincere. These are not separate constructs from *tapas*; sincerity and discipline gradually give rise to courage, strength, and simplicity.
4. *Svadhyaya* refers to self-study or insight. The development of such self-awareness comes through study of the scriptures as well as the clear-eyed observation of our own reality, our spirit of self-exploration.
5. *Ishvara-pranidhana* means to "give to God," or to offer the fruit of ourselves, our work, and our devotion to the God of our own understanding.

Asanas are physical poses. In Hindi and Sanskrit, *asana* literally means "seat," the place where one sits. This guideline describes postures that help to focus the mind and attain a state of balance.

Pranayama refers to the practice that helps us harness our life force. *Prana* means "life energy," and *yama* means "control." *Pranayama* involves the regulation of breath through *puraka* (inhalation), *rechaka* (exhalation), and *kumbhaka* (retention).

Pratyahara is often referred to as sense withdrawal, but it is more than that. It involves an ability to delve deeply within ourselves, where we can reside free from the influences of sensory perception and the external world.

Dharana is concentration. Yoga really begins with paying attention. Concentration merges into meditation, and meditation leads to *samadhi*.

Dhyana means "meditation." In the *dhyana* stage, the act of meditation and the object of meditation remain distinct and separate entities.

Samadhi is the state of complete immersion. Unlike in *dhyana*, there is no distinction between meditator and object. In *samadhi*, we transcend the body and senses and merge with the universal consciousness.

One important thing to understand about the Yoga Sutras—and therefore about Classical Yoga—is that the text presents a dualistic approach to yoga in which matter and spirit are separate from one another. The sutras see the purpose of yoga as transcending matter so spirit can exist in pure form. As long as spirit is bound by matter, it cannot rise. This approach is just one of many; the concept of dualism is not shared by schools that believe in the ultimate unity of spirit and matter in the universal consciousness.

The Postclassical period differs from the Classical period in this way. Postclassical yoga reflects the nondualistic principles of the Vedic period, which derive from the realization that all forms of matter are simply different expressions of the same reality, *brahman*. An interesting development of the Postclassical period was the focus on the body, an aspect that had hitherto been ignored. Yoga practitioners began to view the body in a new light. Instead of a mere receptacle, the body came to be regarded as a temple to be cleansed and cared for.

In Bhakti Flow Yoga, both dualism and nondualism are part of the sacred journey. There is nothing to decide here. There are times in life when we are in survival mode, or moments when we witness death, when we may come from a place of dualism. But nondualism echoes the teachings of oneness and unification. This is the place where we know we are part of the divine, not separate from it. The important thing is to move toward decluttering and clearing the mind to recognize what is in front of us. From there, we simply choose without fear. Again, there really is no -*ism* in Bhakti Flow Yoga.

Hatha Yoga

As a result of the emphasis on physical rejuvenation, the Postclassical period saw the birth of Hatha Yoga, which is what we in the West know simply as "yoga."

Hatha comprises two Sanskrit syllables: *ha* and *tha*. *Ha* is understood to mean the spirit or divine consciousness, the sun, and the incoming breath, whereas *tha* stands for nature, the conscious mind, the moon, and the outgoing breath. Therefore, Hatha Yoga represents the harmonious integration of all these elements, resulting in the development of a steadfast will and balance of mind.

The Pradipika is a seminal text on Hatha Yoga and is understood to have been written by Swami Swatamarama, who lived sometime between the twelfth and fifteenth centuries. The Pradipika consists of four sections:

Section One: *Yamas* (discipline); *niyamas* (observances); asanas, or postures; and diet
Section Two: *Pranayama* (breath control and channeling of energy) and *shatkarmas* (methods of internal cleansing)
Section Three: *Mudras* (gestures of the hand); *bandhas* (internal locks to retain *prana*, or psychic energy, within certain parts of the body); *nadis* (channels through which energy flows); and *kundalini* (evolutionary energy)
Section Four: *Pratyahara* (restraining the senses); *dharana* (mental concentration); *dhyana* (deep contemplation); and *samadhi* (a state of absorption or pure bliss)

Correct practice of Hatha Yoga leads both to a refinement of the body and mind and to harmony between body, mind, and soul or spirit. The Pradipika shows practitioners how to experience Divinity within, how to witness the clear light of a purified consciousness through moral and physical discipline, mental focus, awareness and control of the senses, and insight into their own true nature.

In addition to Hatha Yoga, the Postclassical period gave rise to other important systems, including Tantra Yoga, Kundalini Yoga, Siddha Yoga, and Mantra Yoga. Elements of all four are woven into Bhakti Flow Yoga.

The word *tantra* means "opening out." Tantric Yoga evolved around the concept that blocks or knots at the conscious and subconscious levels prevent us from realizing *shakti* (the dynamic energy of the spirit). Tantra yogis seek to realize *shakti* by dissolving blocks, allowing for the expansion of all aspects of the human consciousness. On a certain level, this is a great way to look at the goal of Bhakti Flow Yoga. Our aim is to clear the blockages in life that prevent us from feeling worthy and connected. Dissolving these blocks helps us find our dharma (duty) and leads us to the ultimate service of others.

Unfortunately, Tantra Yoga has been misinterpreted by many to mean a state of heightened sexuality. This misconception has been fed by the misdeeds of numerous self-styled gurus. But this is not what the practice is truly about. Tantra seeks to establish an awareness of and develop harmony between the male and female aspects inherent in each individual for the purpose of realizing the universe as a manifestation of Shakti, the Mother Goddess or divine energy.

Practitioners of Kundalini Yoga seek to awaken the *kundalini*, the dormant spiritual energy in every human that resides at the base of the spine. When *kundalini* is awakened, it rises through the chakras, or centers of consciousness, to the highest level—the *sahasrara chakra*. At this level, it is said that the yogi realizes *brahman* (the ultimate reality). The yogi merges with divine reality and enters a state of pure bliss.

Siddha Yoga is based on Tantra Yoga. It focuses on turning the awareness inward through meditation so the practitioner may come to truly know the Self. The main practices include meditation, chanting, selfless service, and study.

Mantra Yoga draws on both the Vedas and tantric philosophy. Adherents of this system aspire toward spiritual development and self-actualization through the repetitive chanting of specific mantras, or sound seeds. Such chanting can focus the conscious mind, helping the yogi to minimize stress and relax, and some practitioners consider it to be an easy method of drawing the mind inward.

The period after Postclassical, known as the Modern period, has seen the growth of interest in yoga across the world. In 1893, a young Indian named Swami Vivekananda journeyed to Chicago to speak at the Parliament of Religions. He was the first person from India to influence the American mind with the timeless truth of yoga and Vedanta.

In modern times, many students of Hatha Yoga have gone on to develop their own systems derived from the traditional styles. Creators of new yoga styles base these styles on their own individual understanding of

Hatha Yoga combined with the perceived needs of the societies in which they live, making the evolution of yoga a living, breathing thing.

Vinyasa Yoga, referring to the synchronization of breath and yoga, is the style on which I drew most often in the creation of Bhakti Flow Yoga. Many other schools of yoga, described here, particularly influenced me and Bhakti Flow Yoga.

IYENGAR YOGA

Developed by B. K. S. Iyengar, student and brother-in-law of Sri Krishnamacharya, Iyengar Yoga emphasizes alignment. Students are taught postures in ways that help them develop a high level of precision using props such as blocks, cushions, and other forms of support.

ASHTANGA YOGA

Developed by Pattabhi Jois—who, like Iyengar, was Sri Krishnamacharya's student and brother-in-law—this style is not, as the name may imply, based totally on Patanjali's Ashtanga Yoga. This style is very physical, with an emphasis on synchronizing the breath with a specific set of postures performed in a defined order. The practice generates a lot of heat within the body, typically causing profuse sweating that is said to have a detoxifying effect.

BIKRAM YOGA

Taught by Bikram Choudhury, this style of Hatha Yoga involves twenty-six poses executed in a specific order. The poses are performed in a heated environment, between 100° and 110° F. This type of yoga is suited to those who are energetic, as it requires vigorous physical exertion.

INTEGRAL YOGA

This style was developed by Swami Satchidananda (who chanted OM at Woodstock), one of Swami Sivananda's students. Integral Yoga combines poses, breathing methods, modes of relaxation, and meditation with a view to making the body and mind work in unison. The emphasis is more on function than form.

SIVANANDA YOGA

Based on the teachings of Swami Sivananda, this style of yoga was developed by his student Swami Vishnudevananda. Students of Sivananda Yoga are taught the Sun Salutation (Surya Namaskar) along with a specific sequence of twelve postures, breathing techniques, relaxation poses, and mantra chanting.

JIVAMUKTI YOGA

Introduced by Sharon Gannon and David Life, Jivamukti Yoga is the founders' interpretation of their experience with yoga, as taught by Pattabhi Jois, combined with concepts drawn from spiritual teachings.

This style, found mostly in the United States, aims to teach students how to practice yogic principles in the course of daily life. There is an emphasis on the traditional aspects of yoga such as meditation, chanting, asanas, and study.

POWER YOGA

Based on Ashtanga, Power Yoga incorporates elements of Vinyasa but is a more vigorous style aimed at developing physical fitness and flexibility. This style does not involve adherence to a fixed series of poses as Ashtanga Yoga does.

Encouragingly, the number of modern-day yoga practitioners is increasing. More and more of us are seeking greater harmony, fulfillment, and meaning in our lives and are finding it through yoga. It is important to realize that even the most seemingly physical yoga practice is rooted in the deep and abiding search for truth that has spanned many centuries.

There are many doors into the great living room we call yoga. We all enter in our most authentic and unique way. Some of us go through the door that is clearly marked Physical Practice. There are other doorways marked Meditation, Breathing, Sense Control, and so on. But here is the secret: all of these doors lead us down a corridor of practice that ultimately opens into the same room, where all of the various techniques merge into one lifestyle. We have access to everything, and we can play with every method to see how it works for us.

For me, it is about my intention and whether I am ultimately being of service to others. If not, then my path is to find ways to declutter, unblock, reconsider, and—quite plainly—begin again. If I am not kinder and more open, then it is time to try something different. This big living room has everything I need to find my way home to the heart of the practice.

CHAPTER 3

Nada Yoga

A QUEST FOR THE DIVINE
THROUGH SOUND

For years now, modern scientists have been conducting studies on sound and its impact. Scientific research has revealed what yogis understood thousands of years ago: sound can have a profound effect on matter. Humans, animals, and even inanimate objects are influenced by sound. Experiments conducted over several years by the Swiss scientist and medical practitioner Hans Jenny demonstrated that different vibratory frequencies have varying effects on certain substances. In Jenny's experiments, vibrations from a sound such as OH, which has a low pitch, caused a substance to form a circle, whereas the high-frequency sound OM produced an outline similar to the *shri yantra*, the symbol that represents OM. Jenny also found that the higher the frequency, the more intricate the form. Based on his experiments, he concluded that sound creates form, the fundamental truth that yogis discovered millennia ago.*

Chanting and mantra are an important part of Bhakti Flow Yoga. The understanding that sound has the power to influence consciousness, leading to purification and ultimate union with the divine, is fundamental to Bhakti Yoga as well as to Bhakti Flow. Chanting is a vehicle for connecting to something deeper than ourselves, and it is widely acknowledged that chanting has the power to soothe troubled minds. This belief has a scientific basis, as demonstrated by the experiments of the French physician Alfred Tomatis. His research found that many sacred chants of diverse cultural origins have high vibratory frequencies (3,000 Hz and higher) that activate the cerebral cortex, affecting memory, thinking, and spatial ability.

---

*Hans Jenny, *Cymatics: The Structure and Dynamics of Waves and Vibrations* (Basel, Switzerland: Basilius, 1967).

I have always been drawn to spiritual music. It isn't so much the lyrics, but the warmth my heart feels while I'm singing. Singing has always come naturally for me. I grew up with parents and siblings who loved music. We sang all the time. We sang in church. We sang for no good reason at all. Our house was filled with song. When I went off to college, my mom said that what she missed most was me singing around the house. My parents have left this world, but their voices stay with me, their favorite songs etched in my life forever. Even as my mother passed away, I was able to sing back to her the very songs she sang to me when I was young. Is there a kinder gift our creator could have given at a moment like that? I don't think so.

Later in life, after a break with the religion I'd known since childhood, I was lost about where to allow sacred sound to live in my life. When I discovered Bhakti Yoga (or more likely, when it discovered me), I was so very happy. Now I sing mostly because I can. I sing because I have been given a voice, one that will not last forever. I sing because it is truth and it is refuge and it is devotion and it is playfulness and it is home. I sing with others because it reminds us that we are here together, if only for a while.

In India, *japa* (chanting mantras to oneself) is of Vedic origin. The word *mantra* derives from *man* ("to ponder") and *tra*, which refers to a thing's instrumental nature. A mantra, then, is like a device that enables you to think deeply, focus on your consciousness, and work toward purifying this consciousness. Mantras can be chanted aloud, meditated on in silence, whispered, or visualized. Silent mantras are known as *ajapa*.

All mantras derive from the Sanskrit alphabet. They can comprise a letter, a syllable, a group of syllables, a word, or a collection of words. For a mantra to be effective, it needs to be passed down from a guru who is spiritually advanced, so that the mantra is infused with that person's positive vibrations.

According to yogic thought, we are each a mass of vibrations; our experience of life derives from our internal vibratory frequencies. When *prana* (energy) flows smoothly through us, our minds and bodies function harmoniously, in tune with the natural rhythm. Thousands of years ago in India, yogis discovered that vocal sounds vibrate through the entire body, and chants composed of syllables or words with the right frequencies help resolve the body's vibratory imbalances and enable *prana* to flow freely through the chakras.

Sound reverberates beyond the obvious; there is more to it than what we normally hear in the course of our daily lives. The ancient yogis believed that sound can ultimately lead to the transformation of the consciousness. It is in this belief that Nada Yoga, the Yoga of Sound, has its origins.

The Practice of Nada Yoga

Nada Yoga is the ancient Indian science of sound. The word *nada* comes from the Sanskrit *nad*, meaning "flow." Literally, *nada* refers to the continuous flow of consciousness; more generally, it is understood to mean "sound." The ancient yogis believed that the entire universe was created by and is permeated with the same primordial sound. It is this original vibration—the *shabda brahman* (supreme sound)—that lies at the root of all phenomena. All other sounds manifest from this.

The science of Nada Yoga explores the nature of sound, both audible and inaudible, and how it influences consciousness. Listening helps to calm and focus the mind. It is only with a tranquil mind that we can realistically work toward physical, mental, and spiritual harmony. Nada Yoga aims to purify the consciousness through the development of equanimous awareness of sound.

At the start of some classes, especially our more beginner-friendly ones, I will often ask students to come to a comfortable sitting position and close their eyes. I ask them to take in the immediate sounds around them. What do they hear right away? What do they think or feel about those sounds? I ask them to notice the sounds nearest to them—the sound of the floor as someone is walking in, a mat being rolled out, or even the sound of my voice. From there, I ask that they "stretch" their hearing to take in the sounds just outside the practice space, perhaps noticing voices in the lobby and eventually the activity sounds in the street just outside. Can they hear the tree branches brushing against the windows, the buses and cars, and all the sounds of urban dwelling? Then I ask that they stretch their hearing as far as possible. Can they hear across the city all the way to the ocean and beyond? (Okay, that may be a stretch, but in and of itself, it is a powerful exercise.)

This exercise leads us from hearing (the simple act of perceiving sound) to active listening (which requires conscious choice and leads to learning). As we begin to listen to the farthest sounds, we also have the opportunity to notice any feelings or thoughts that arise about those sounds. Some sounds spark certain emotions. Some we tend to push away, while others we try to linger with as long as possible. Some sounds have us sticking with them while we create stories about them. And there are some toward which we are absolutely neutral. All of these reactions are perfectly fine. Noticing the reactions, even the neutral ones, is what's most interesting in this exercise.

Once we stretch our hearing as far outward as possible, we slowly turn this around and carefully come back home, picking up sounds we may not have heard on the outward journey. As we draw our listening back into the practice space, the experience can become much more intimate and personal. We can hear and listen to our breath. From there, we can listen so carefully that we detect the beat of our heart. I ask students to stay with this until they can hear the very sound of their blood flowing. When we get to this moment in the meditation on sound, I ask that students listen carefully to their blood until they detect the presence of the same blood that flowed in their parents, their grandparents, and all through their ancestors, allowing a comfort to set in, knowing that there really was never a time we did not exist on some level. It is then that I ask them to try and remember the beginning of time itself and how there was actually a time when there was absolutely nothing. It is said that from this nothingness a vibration occurred, and from that vibration, sound was born. From there, we join voices to create the sound of OM.

Sound can be external or internal. External sound (*ahata nada*) is produced when two or more objects come into contact with each other. This sound is experienced at the sensory level. Music, traffic, and other environmental noises are all *ahata nada*, clearly audible to the ordinary ear. Internal sounds (*anahata nada*) are the result of inner vibrations and can be heard only by those who are trained to listen. Also known as "unstruck sounds," internal sounds are not created by external objects but are manifestations of the subtle vibrations of *prana*. *Anahata nada* is the sound of silence. In training our minds to listen to silence, we actively involve our consciousness and gradually develop insight.

In India, the earliest known acknowledgment of the divine power of sound can be found in the Vedas. The concept of awakening the human consciousness through *shabda* (the Word) is of Vedic origin. Through their personal experience of the divine sound, the mystics of the Vedic age realized that specific words or sounds can help draw the senses inward, allowing the seeker to tune in to his or her internal vibrations and, in so doing, work toward spiritual awakening. Mantra recitation is believed to have originated during this time. Some refer to this phase of Nada Yoga as Shabda Yoga.

As with followers of other paths of yoga, the supreme quest of the Nada yogi is union with the divine Self, a state of total silence and bliss. In Nada Yoga, this ultimate sound of silence is known as the *para nada*, the root source of all sounds. *Para*, meaning "beyond," denotes the highest state of consciousness, the unconditioned mind. This transcendent sound, which is nonsensory, has the highest frequency and can be experienced only by someone who has risen above the sphere of the senses. Sounds that vibrate at very high frequencies are inaudible at a sensory level. This is why the *para nada* is known as the sound of silence and can be perceived only in deep meditation.

According to the Upanishads, OM is *para nada*. This OM is not the audible mantra that people chant, which is created and perceived by the senses. It is a transcendent OM that is still and eternal. It is the divine basis of existence, the pure and primordial sound from which all matter originates. The entire universe resonates with and is sustained by this vibration. Inaudible on the sensory plane, it is perceived by the receptive mind. In Nada Yoga, sounds that are perceived by the mind rather than by the ear's sensory capacity are known as *pashyanti nada* (visualized sounds). *Pashyanti nada* are those that we hear in our dreams, sounds that spring from the subconscious. These sounds, heard when we are in a deep state of contemplation and oblivious of the external world, have a lower frequency than *para nada*. In deep states of contemplation, external sounds do not reach the yogi; he or she hears only inner sounds that are unlike ordinary environmental sounds.

Sounds at a lower level than *pashyanti* but finer than those that are clearly audible are coarse noises; they are categorized as *madhyama*, meaning "in the middle." Intermediate sounds that are barely audible, such as whispering, are *madhyama nada*. These sounds are relatively subtle but have fewer vibrations than *para* and *pashyanti nada*.

At the lowest level of nada are *vaikhari* (ordinary sounds). These have the lowest frequency and are produced physically when one object comes into contact with another. Chimes, drumbeats, the spoken word, and clapping all belong to the category of *vaikhari nada*.

The Nada yogi experiences the universe as a mass of vibrations. In Nada Yoga, the quest for divine truth or the pure Self takes practitioners along the path of sound. First, the yogi learns to listen, to actively observe all sounds without reacting. Absorption in sound, even if it is only for a few minutes every day, helps to calm and focus the mind. By learning to experience all sounds —pleasant and unpleasant—with equanimity, the Nada yogi gradually refines his or her consciousness. As the yogi's stock of ignorance, craving, and aversion slowly depletes, the mind rises above conditioning. Bit by bit, the yogi becomes conscious of subtle inner sounds.

To experience *para nada*, the practitioner needs to begin by actively listening to coarse sounds. As the yogi progresses to higher levels of consciousness, finer sounds become more apparent. What the ordinary ear perceives as stillness is actually buzzing with sounds that a mind capable of listening to silence can hear.

The Bhakti yogi's approach to sound involves the recitation of mantras, whether repeated to oneself or in company with others (*kirtan*). *Kirtan* is typically a call-and-response activity and can be both moving and meditative.

Initially, the focus in Bhakti Yoga is on the audible, or *vaikhari*, sound of the mantra, warming up to receive the *madhyama* sound. The yogi then proceeds to muttering or whispering the mantra, aspiring to merge with it. A stage comes when the lips stop moving and the yogi's awareness of the mantra, the object of devotion, evolves from sensory to mental. Some call this the *upanshu* stage.

As the mind becomes calmer, the yogi begins to think the mantra or repeat it silently in his or her consciousness. The mind becomes absorbed in the vibration of the mantra, tuning in to its subtle rhythm and becoming aware of inner sounds in the process. For the Bhakti yogi, it is as if the mind is singing to the Beloved. At this point, also known as the *manasika* stage, the focus is internal. As the practice develops, there comes a stage when the yogi no longer needs to recite or think the mantra consciously; rather, it arises from within. The yogi listens, enraptured, as the music plays by itself. Awareness of sounds such as these is known as *ajapa japa*. At this point, no effort is required to create a sound; the sound simply exists. It has become part of the yogi's nature.

As practitioners become more aware of inner noises and more oblivi-ous of external ones, they approach the stage of *pratyahara*. The ability to listen to fine, inaudible sounds increases. With regular and sincere prac-tice, the sound of the mantra gradually transforms into a constant, uni-form sound—*nada*.

In Bhakti Yoga, as with Bhakti Flow, an integral part of the experience is fostering a deep awareness of sound and, through this awareness, find-ing a connection to the Creator and all of creation. This is one reason we chant in Bhakti Flow, and it is a key reason why we learn to truly listen. These songs are lullabies to and from the Beloved. The end result of this practice often allows us to come to a place of pure quiet and connectivity, and from this place, the stage is set for true listening to begin.

The technique of Nada Yoga has been handed down from guru, or teacher, to *shishya* (pupil) since its inception. It is advisable for aspirants to practice Nada Yoga under expert guidance. The Nada yogi also needs to develop the right attitude and be careful about diet.

In general, experienced teachers and practitioners of Nada Yoga rec-ommend soothing, positive music for those who are taking their first steps on this path. It is best if the music is instrumental, because words can often distract the mind.

An interesting note is that Indian classical musicians of the past were required to practice yoga, particularly *pranayama* practices such as Bhra-mari (Humming Breath), and also had to learn to listen to *anahata nada* to refine their perception of sound. *Dhrupad*, one of the oldest styles of Hin-dustani classical music, is infused with a spiritual quality and was originally performed within temple precincts by priests as an offering to the divine. Listening to traditional Indian music such as *ragas*, *slokas*, *talas*, mantras, and *bhajans* helps to relieve stress, offering a few moments of peace amid the hurly-burly of modern living.

Nada Yoga teaches us to listen beyond the sensory plane. Over time and with regular practice, the need for external music recedes, and the Nada yogi is able to meditate on his or her own inner music.

A Few Moments of Quiet in Modern Life

Sound can help you find the stillness that is so hard to come by in your daily life. Listening to calming music for a few minutes every day relaxes the mind and is a good way to begin your practice of Nada Yoga. Ini-tially, the music you select should have an even tenor to help you focus. Frequent and wide variations in pitch and emotion are not suitable for contemplation. In general, I recommend repetitive sounds that bring you to a calm state yet do not induce sleep. Contemplation should be a wakeful experience. Sounds with a transfixing but not hypnotic pulse are encouraged.

Even spending fifteen minutes twice a day listening in a contempla-tive state can make a positive difference. Meditating on sound relieves stress and induces feelings of tranquility and joy. Over time, with disciplined practice, this form of meditation can help you evolve spiritually. The seers of old, in their wisdom, discovered that a deep understanding of sound or vibration can lead to knowledge of oneself. The essence of this practice lies in the development of equanimity. Relax and focus on the music without reacting to it. Initially, you may find it hard to listen without liking or disliking the sounds, but as you establish awareness, you will gradually learn to observe sound from a balanced perspective. Try listening to the same music every day, preferably at the same time, in full concentration. Eventually, you may become aware of subtle inner sounds. Focus on these sounds when they arise, meditating on them rather than on the external music.

There will come a time when you will be able to meditate without the aid of music. Continue your meditation regularly, listening to your own inner music.

CHAPTER 4

Energy, Pranayama, and Meditation

ENERGY IS KEY IN OUR LIVES. It powers us, and how well we function depends on the quality and use of the energy we have. The quality of energy, in turn, relies on the state of consciousness. This is something we have all experienced. Think about how you feel good around some people but not so good around others. Or how you can sense positive or negative energies emanating from different people. Our state of mind determines the nature of the energy we put into the world.

Not long ago, I was brought down by an illness that had me near death's door. Everyone around me thought my time was nearly done. Even I felt my life force quickly slipping away. But there was a moment when I decided not to give in, to use the little bit of energy I had to reawaken and return to the living. In that moment, I used my slightest bit of breath to carefully awaken my body, my mind, and my heart.

It took everything I had to move my body, then eventually to stand up, and then to take a step forward. That step gave me the hope to take another. At first everything hurt. Tears were a regular part of my daily growth and return to vibrant health.

The months it took to restore my health reflected a daily exercise involving intense study of how and where I used energy, how I manufactured and even wasted it, and how I could conserve and store it. The obvious and overt actions came from my conscious decisions. *Everything* originated from my choosing to try.

My greatest lesson has been the appreciation of the energy I have and the recognition that I have only a certain amount to spend within this gift of life. As a result, I am careful now to use it wisely, especially in my relationships. There are no more trivialities. Wasted energy is wasted life, and we will never get it back. With a joyful heart, I embrace with great gratitude whatever remains.

In yoga, *prana* (energy) is of central importance. Every living organism is infused with *prana*, the nature of which is universal. The flow of *prana* affects the way we think, feel, and act. One of the principles espoused by yogic science is that the regulation of energy can be used to bring about transformation. In other words, it's possible to enhance mental, emotional, and physical function by first understanding how energy works and then putting that understanding into practice to actively manage and drive energy.

The balanced flow of *prana* helps yogis ascend to the realization of pure-state awareness as the ultimate truth. Bhakti Flow Yoga, along with Hatha Yoga, aims to invigorate the flow of *prana* and remove obstructions to the free flow of energy.

Prana and Pranayama

> Inhale and God approaches you.
> Hold the inhalation, and God remains with you.
> Exhale, and you approach God.
> Hold the exhalation, and surrender to God.
>
> — KRISHNAMACHARYA

Breath is a mirror of the mind. The way we breathe can both indicate and directly impact how we feel. Subtle, regular breathing reflects a calm state of mind, whereas heavy, coarse, rapid respiration speaks of an agitated mind.

Pranayama comes from the Sanskrit words *prana* (life force) and *ayama* (control). Translated literally, *pranayama* means "breath control," but the practice is deeper than that. It is more of a holistic approach that involves purifying, balancing, and regulating the flow of *prana*. We can harness energy positively through the consistent and scientific practice of *pranayama*, which aids in the development of consciousness by establishing harmony between *prana* and the mind. Ancient yogis understood this, and they developed breathing techniques that focus and direct *prana* to propel the practitioner to higher levels of consciousness.

Here are some basic *pranayama* techniques commonly used in Bhakti Flow Yoga:

- Kapalabhati Pranayama (Cleansing Breath): A quick, strong breath involving passive inhalations and short, powerful exhalations. This breath helps to eliminate stress and negative emotions. It also promotes good digestion and circulation.
- Anuloma Viloma or Nadi Shodhana (Alternate Nostril Breathing): An easy *pranayama* that involves inhaling through one nostril and exhaling through the other. This helps to cleanse the respiratory system,

improve concentration and memory, and prepare students for the practice of other *pranayamas*.

- Ujjayi Pranayama (Victorious Breath): Because this makes a sound like an ocean roaring, it is often called Ocean Breath. The back of the throat is constricted while breathing, generating the "ocean in the distance" sound. Ujjayi can help you concentrate, increase awareness, and generate internal heat. This breath is often used during Vinyasa Yoga practices.

Though the practice of *pranayama* can improve the state of both mind and body, you should practice it with care. The right approach is to train under a certified expert and consult a physician about the suitability of each *pranayama* for your individual health conditions.

The Kosha Concept

Translated roughly, *kosha* means "sheath" or "layer." According to yogic thought, five different layers cover the incorruptible Self (*atman*). In Vedanta philosophy, these *koshas* constitute the nonself (as distinct from the incorruptible Self); to realize the incorruptible Self, one must journey inward through each *kosha* from the gross to the subtle.

Being alive is a many-layered experience. It is an expression of our physical, cerebral, emotional, and spiritual states of being. Each of us lives differently, but at the core, we are the same, an embodiment of the ultimate truth. This divine part of us is hidden by *maya* (the veil of illusion).

Maya makes us perceive things as other than what they really are. Each *kosha* refers to a specific type of *maya*, or appearance. The five *koshas* are as follows:

> *Annamaya kosha*
> *Pranamaya kosha*
> *Manomaya kosha*
> *Vijnanamaya kosha*
> *Anandamaya kosha*

Annamaya kosha takes its name from the Sanskrit word *anna*, meaning "food." The term refers to our physical being, the aspect that we can touch and feel every waking moment. Of all five layers, this is the most tangible. The practice of yoga involves nurturing the body as well as understanding it from a spiritual perspective. This helps us live better, both externally and internally. As we begin to recognize that the physical aspect of our being is an impermanent, constantly changing entity, we gradually develop a sense of detachment that enables us to progress inward during meditation.

Pranamaya kosha is the next level of being. *Prana*, as we know, refers to the vital life force that manifests as breath and flows through the body.

We cannot see the *pranamaya kosha*, but we can feel it in the vibrations of our breath. Whether or not *prana* flows smoothly and evenly through our entire being depends on the balance between mind, body, and spirit. The practice of *pranayama* helps regulate and direct *prana*.

Manomaya kosha comes from *manas* (mind) and oversees the function of the body and breath. Physically, the brain, spinal cord, nerves, and sensory faculties constitute this kosha, and it finds expression in our thoughts, feelings, and responses. It is associated with our sense of attachment and possession and of being different from others.

Vijnanamaya kosha corresponds to ego and intellect. The word *vijnana* means "to know deeply or intensely." It manifests as wisdom, not just intellectual knowledge, enabling introspection and the development of insight. The clearer our awareness of this level of being, the more developed our faculty of discernment. We begin to see things as they really are, not as they appear to be. Serious meditation helps us penetrate the *vijnanamaya kosha*.

Anandamaya kosha is the innermost and most subtle layer. This is the *kosha* that surrounds the *atman*. The word *ananda* means "bliss." However, this is not the bliss associated with sensory pleasure and experienced at the mundane level. It is independent of emotion, sensory stimuli, and thought. Awareness of the *anandamaya kosha* manifests as a state of total contentment, peace, and joy, even if it lasts just a few moments. It is said that we experience this state fully in the state of deep sleep.

It is when we transcend the subtle sheath of *anandamaya kosha* that we realize *atman*. While the five *koshas* are changeable, the Self is unchanging.

Chakras

Chakras are centers of consciousness in the subtle body, invisible because they are formless. In Sanskrit, *chakra* literally means "wheel." The chakras, located along the spine, are always in motion. These currents of energy whirl around, transmitting *prana* to different parts of the body as well as to the mind. Awakened chakras move in a clockwise direction, helping to restore and maintain inner balance.

These spinning wheels of energy can be powerful. It is possible to harness their potential only when obstructions disappear and energy flows freely. Hindrances to the flow of *prana* upset the balance within and between the chakras, leading to physical, emotional, and mental disturbances and blocking spiritual growth. The practice of yoga helps to clear each chakra, unleashing its true power in the process.

There are seven chakras, each of which is associated with specific immutable qualities. Depending on the state of our consciousness, these qualities may be latent or developed. They begin to manifest with the awakening and ascent of *kundalini*, the spiritual force present in each human being. As we grow in meditation, *kundalini* unfolds, progressively activating the various chakras and allowing their qualities to find expression.

THE SEVEN CHAKRAS

Muladhara is the first, or root, chakra and is located at the base of the spine below the sacrum. Its quality is innocence, what little children express so spontaneously. Innocence enables us to know pure, unconditional happiness. We sometimes see this in the gentle look or smile of an adult. But more often than not, the passage to adulthood robs us of direct knowledge of innocence, although we never truly lose its inherent presence within us. This is one of the qualities that becomes reawakened during our spiritual development.

Here are the characteristics of the *muladhara* chakra:

- *Location:* Base of the spine, in the groin area (This chakra is positioned at the source of *kundalini.*)
- *Anatomical significance:* Influences the function of kidneys, blood, muscles, and adrenal glands
- *Color:* Red
- *Symbol:* A square within a circle ringed by four lotus petals

The second, or sacral, chakra is the *swadisthana*, which is associated with creative potential, concentration, and spiritual knowledge that transcends the intellect. People in whom the *swadisthana* chakra is activated tend to be more focused and aware of both inner and outer reality, being able to sense subtle vibrations in the body as well as in the world around them.

Here are the characteristics of the *swadisthana* chakra:

- *Location:* Lower abdomen, in the vicinity of the genitals
- *Anatomical significance:* Influences the health of the stomach and reproductive organs
- *Color:* Orange
- *Symbol:* Either five or six lotus petals around a circle

The inherent qualities of the third chakra—known as the *manipura*, or solar plexus, chakra—are generosity and contentment. A clear *manipura* chakra helps us conquer stress and also promotes peace of mind. When *kundalini* rises through this chakra, we develop a strong sense of morality and spiritual motivation, becoming more balanced as energy flows freely.

Here are the characteristics of the *manipura* chakra:

- *Location:* Below the diaphragm, halfway between the rib cage and the navel
- *Anatomical significance:* Influences the function of the nervous system, digestive system, liver, pancreas, spleen, and gall bladder
- *Color:* Yellow
- *Symbol:* Ten lotus petals around a circle with a triangle inside it

The fourth chakra is the *anahata*, or heart, chakra; it is the abode of the Self, or divine consciousness. Many of us pass from one life to another, unaware of the spirit or pure consciousness present within us that nothing can tarnish. Spiritual awakening alone helps us to experience the power, freedom, and pure joy of the divine Self. As the energy in this chakra begins to flow freely, we gradually rise above ego and conditioning, drawing closer to our true selves and emanating love, compassion, and goodwill toward others.

Here are the characteristics of the *anahata* chakra:

- *Location:* At the sternum, around the center of the breastbone
- *Anatomical significance:* Influences the health of the lungs, heart, thymus gland, and circulatory system
- *Colors:* Pink and green
- *Symbol:* A six-pointed star within a circle ringed by twelve lotus petals

The *vishuddha*, or throat, chakra is the fifth chakra and is associated with the quality of detachment. As *kundalini* ascends through this chakra, compassion grows, relationships improve, and feelings of remorse and guilt gradually dissolve. We develop an awareness of our oneness with the universe.

Here are the characteristics of the *vishuddha* chakra:

- *Location:* Throat
- *Anatomical significance:* Influences the function of the thyroid gland, lungs, and entire respiratory system
- *Colors:* Light blue and turquoise
- *Symbol:* A circle within a circle ringed by sixteen lotus petals, or a circle enclosing a triangle

Forgiveness and empathy are the qualities inherent to the sixth chakra, known as the *ajna*, or third eye, chakra. As energy begins to flow freely in this chakra, feelings of hurt, resentment, anger, and animosity weaken, giving rise to tolerance, understanding, humility, and nobility. We gradually become more altruistic.

Here are the characteristics of the *ajna* chakra:

- *Location:* Between the eyes, in the center of the forehead
- *Anatomical significance:* Influences the condition of the pituitary gland, eyes, ears, nose, and bones
- *Color:* Indigo
- *Symbol:* A circle with two large lotus petals on each side and a triangle within

The final stage in the evolution of consciousness occurs at the *sahasrara*, or crown, chakra. The qualities of all the other chakras come together in the seventh. When this chakra is awakened, we directly experience ultimate reality.

Here are the characteristics of the *sahasrara* chakra:

- *Location:* Above the head
- *Anatomical significance:* Associated with the health of the brain, pineal gland, and central nervous system
- *Color:* Violet
- *Symbol:* A lotus with a thousand petals

Nadis

Nadis (channels) are the subtle energy conduits within the body through which *prana* flows. They do not have a physical form and are invisible to the average eye; however, developed yogis can see their formless presence. *Nadi* is a derivative of the Sanskrit word *nad,* which means "flow." Just as an efficient irrigation system keeps fields well hydrated and crops nourished, so does a network of clean and strong *nadis* enable *prana* to flow freely, leading to mental, emotional, and physical well-being. Of the tens of thousands of *nadis* each person has, the *ida, pingala,* and *sushumna nadis* are considered the most important.

The *sushumna nadi* is the central *nadi,* running from the base of the spine to the top of the head and passing through all seven chakras as it progresses upward. This is the channel through which *kundalini* rises when awakened.

The *ida* and *pingala nadis* twirl around the *sushumna nadi* from top to bottom, intersecting at each chakra. *Ida* begins and ends on the left of *sushumna; pingala* begins and ends on the right. All three *nadis* finally meet at the *ajna* chakra between the eyebrows.

The *ida* and *pingala nadis* are each associated with distinct characteristics. All that is cool, feminine, and supportive in us derives from *ida,* which is often identified as the lunar *nadi* and visualized as being white or blue. *Ida* directs our mental function. *Pingala,* often identified as the sun or solar *nadi,* reflects the warm, motivating, and masculine aspects of human nature and controls our physical processes. It is represented by the color red.

How *ida* and *pingala* function and work together determines the state of our physical, mental, and spiritual development. The two *nadis* alternate dominance throughout the day. However, one of them tends to have more frequent and longer periods of ascendancy in each of us, making that *nadi* more influential in our being. Ida dominates in some people, making them more calm, thoughtful, introspective, and caring but less energetic. In contrast, individuals characterized by strong *pingala* brim with vitality and tend to be creative but not as calm and nurturing as *ida*-dominant people.

Harmonizing *ida* and *pingala* helps to address imbalances in mental, emotional, physical, and spiritual development. Observing Hatha Yoga guidelines and practicing asanas leads to purification and control of the *ida* and *pingala nadis,* thereby resolving the imbalance between them. By aiming to cleanse, regulate, and strengthen these *nadis*, Hatha Yoga enhances the flow of *prana*, letting us realize the potential of our life force.

According to some facets of yogic thought, *sushumna* will not open unless *ida* and *pingala* are in perfect equilibrium. Since *kundalini* can rise only through the *sushumna nadi*, achieving a balance between *ida* and *pingala* is essential for the awakening of *kundalini* and allowing the yogi to progress to higher levels of consciousness.

According to Hatha Yoga teachings, Nadi Shodhana Pranayama (Alternate Nostril Breathing) effectively cleanses *ida* and *pingala*, eventually bringing them into balance. The underlying concept is that *ida* is connected to the left nostril and *pingala* to the right. Breathing through alternate nostrils helps remove obstructions in both *nadis*, thereby facilitating a balanced flow of energy through both.

We can ascertain which *nadi* is dominant at any given time by observing our breath carefully. When breath flows more freely through the left nostril than the right, *ida* is dominant. If it is the other way around, *pingala* is dominant. Asana practice can be planned according to the strength of *ida* and *pingala* at any given time. If *ida* is ascendant, performing vigorous, heat-generating asanas helps to invigorate *pingala*, whereas if *pingala* dominates, *ida* can be energized by practicing asanas that help to focus and calm the mind.

The level of *ida* or *pingala* is indicated by our state of mind as well. When *ida* dominates, we are calm, thoughtful, focused, or even drowsy. *Ida* prevails while we are asleep. A dominant *pingala*, on the other hand, makes us active, enthusiastic, or agitated. A relatively even flow of air through both nostrils helps us to maintain a balance between physical, emotional, and mental orientation of both *nadis*.

As we know, the process of taking control of our energy is holistic, not just through asanas and *pranayama* techniques. Conduct, diet, and lifestyle all play a part in establishing harmony between *ida* and *pingala*. Making a conscious effort to be better than we were yesterday, to be more truthful, loving, and compassionate, to be less resentful and covetous, and to refrain from harming others can go a long way in restoring balance and instilling our lives with the meaning we want.

Bandhas

In yoga, the term *bandha* is used to refer to neuromuscular restraints or locks that prevent *prana* from dissipating or flowing outward. In general, energy does not flow freely and uniformly within the body because of physical, emotional, or mental imbalances. Clearing and regulating the flow of *prana* helps to resolve these problems and facilitate the process of spiritual development.

In the average person, certain parts of the body receive excess energy, whereas other parts don't get enough. Right now, stop and notice any areas of your body that have long forgotten the breath and take a moment to breathe space into them. Observe how it feels.

Uneven *prana* flow and stagnation causes physical as well as psychological disorders. *Bandhas* are employed to contain *prana* in a specific anatomical region for a certain length of time. In effect, *bandha* practice locks the life force in a particular area with a view to regulating blood circulation and revitalizing specific organs. If practiced correctly, *bandhas* help retard the process of oxidation, strengthen the nervous system, improve the function of certain organs, and reinvigorate the individual.

Yogic texts generally tend to focus on three main *bandhas*: Jalandhara Bandha (Chin Lock), Uddiyana Bandha (Abdominal Lock, or Fly-up), and Mula Bandha (Root Lock). The practice of all three *bandhas* together is known as Maha Bandha (Great Lock) or Trayam Bandha (Triple Lock).

In yoga therapy, regular practice of all three *bandhas* is recommended for the health of the digestive and intestinal systems as well as for the prevention of lung and heart ailments. The two *bandhas* used most often in Vinyasa Yoga and during a typical Bhakti Flow Yoga class are Uddiyana and Mula Bandha. As in the case of asanas, *bandhas* need to be practiced under the supervision of a trained and reputable yoga instructor after consultation with your physician.

Especially when practicing Vinyasa Yoga, the use of *bandhas* helps me feel a lightness that allows a seamless flow from pose to pose. Jumping forward and back and moving from standing to sitting, the movements become uniquely connected. Great sages of yore described the activation of *bandhas* as an assist in levitation. Although I have felt a lightness in my flow-based yoga, I have yet to lift so high as to bump my head on the ceiling. However, there's always tomorrow's practice!

JALANDHARA BANDHA

Jal means "net" or "mesh" and refers to the network of *nadis. Dhar* means "to hold or restrain." This *bandha* clears confusion, calms the mind, and relieves anger and stress.

Engaging Jalandhara Bandha causes excess blood to flow out of the organs in the head and neck region, thereby regulating blood circulation and helping to relieve physical ailments such as eye strain and migraines.

Here are the main characteristics of Jalandhara Bandha:

- *Location:* Throat
- *Technique:* Usually performed during Thunderbolt Pose (Vajrasana) or Lotus Pose (Padmasana). Inhale deeply and hold the breath while bowing your head forward, locking your chin between your collarbones. Your arms should be straight and your shoulders raised and thrust forward. Hold this lock as long as it is comfortable. Release by relaxing your shoulders, raising your chin, bringing your head level, and exhaling.

- *Direction of flow:* Regulates the flow of blood and *prana* to your head, heart, and endocrine glands in the neck, draining the area of excess blood. It also prevents *prana* from flowing down from the *sahasrara* chakra and facilitates the free flow of *prana* from the base of your neck to the crown of your head.
- *Anatomical significance:* Affects your pineal, pituitary, thymus, thyroid, and parathyroid glands

UDDIYANA BANDHA

This *bandha* involves exercising the muscles of the abdomen and diaphragm, causing *prana* to flow upward from the belly to the thoracic region. Uddiyana Bandha helps to stimulate the *manipura* chakra. It strengthens the diaphragm, tones the pancreas and spleen, and clears a clogged liver. Its practice is often recommended for relieving constipation.

Here are the main characteristics of Uddiyana Bandha:

- *Location:* Abdomen and diaphragm
- *Technique:* Normally performed in a standing or sitting pose and between an exhalation and an inhalation. Breathing through your nose, inhale fully. On a strong exhalation through your nose, empty your lungs and contract your abdomen. Then relax your abdomen and expand your chest as if you were inhaling again. This sensation should draw your abdominal muscles and organs up, as though you were drawing your navel up your spine. At this point, activate Jalandhara Bandha. Hold for 15 to 30 seconds and repeat three or more times.
- *Direction of flow:* From the abdomen to the thorax
- *Anatomical significance:* Influences the health of the adrenal glands and pancreas

MULA BANDHA

The practice of Mula Bandha exercises the muscles in the pelvic region. This *bandha* helps to resolve psychological and neurotic imbalances that result from sexual frustration or dissatisfaction. Physically, it calms the central and sympathetic nerves and regulates blood flow to the ovaries and the prostate gland, helping to prevent disorders in the urogenital region. Regular and correct practice of this *bandha* tones the bladder, kidneys, and female sex organs. It is also believed to activate the *muladhara* chakra.

Here are the main characteristics of Mula Bandha:

- *Location:* Perineum and cervix
- *Technique:* Sit in Thunderbolt Pose (Vajrasana) or Lotus Pose (Padmasana), inhale deeply, and contract the muscles of your perineum, drawing them upward while holding the breath. The lock tightens these muscles and can be held as long as it is comfortably possible. Release by relaxing the muscles and then exhaling slowly.

- *Direction of flow:* Works with *apana,* or the energy that directs the expulsion of metabolic waste from the *muladhara* chakra down
- *Anatomical significance:* Influences the function of the gonads and perineal glands

Meditation: The Quest for Spiritual Union

The greatest challenge confronting humans today is the same as it was thousands of years ago. It is the quest for stillness within, what Arjuna in the Bhagavad Gita called "the stillness of divine union." A still mind is totally at peace and can withstand the most turbulent of storms.

> The practice of meditation frees one from
> all affliction. This is the path of yoga. Follow it
> with determination and sustained enthusiasm.
>
> — BHAGAVAD GITA (6:23)

When I first came to the practice of meditation, I hadn't a clue what I was supposed to be doing. It seemed like the exercise was designed as a form of self-punishment. I knew to try and sit up straight, not to fidget, and not to speak. At one point, it reminded me of the early days of my parochial education.

I have always been great at fidgeting. In fact, I'm certain that if there were ever an award given out for best fidgeter, I would earn the title. As a kid, I found many ways to control that urge, especially at school or in church. Otherwise, I was always being told to sit up straight and stop moving around so much. By sheer obedience, I learned how to occupy my mind to keep my body still—and consequently kept the powers that be convinced that I was behaving properly. Little did they know that I was merely on a mental holiday, immersed in the fantastical imaginings of a young boy escaping a very small town.

Eventually, I moved from my very small town to a bigger small town, where I noticed a *zendo* at a busy intersection. I walked by it a number of times before I actually stepped in. I didn't really know much about Zen, other than bits I'd learned from several books I'd read. My favorites were by the Dutch author Janwillem van de Wetering, who had spent time in a Zen monastery. His work inspired me to ponder concepts I'd never before imagined. I was intrigued.

The first few visits were a bit excruciating. I sat down and literally felt like I did nothing but wait (painfully!) for the hour to be over. Just getting through that experience made me feel successful. After a few more sits, I began reckoning with my own fluctuations of mind. It was terribly difficult, but I knew it was important and somehow imperative for me to crack through and find those glimpses of nothingness I had read about in Mr. van de Wetering's works.

This is how I learned to commit not simply to the practice of sitting still, but also to the practice of training my mind to listen. At first I wasn't even sure what I was supposed to be listening *for*, but eventually the truth of meditation found me. There is no "listening for." There is just the listening itself, without expectation; a letting go of preconceived notions and limitations, even beyond whatever discomforts arise. My attachments and avoidances became my teachers.

One of my favorite lessons from this period came from a teacher at the *zendo*. He must have noticed the furrow in my brow or the cringe somewhere in my body each time a bus would pull up at the stop outside our center. It was loud: the screeching brakes, the opening and closing of doors, the conversations, the bus pulling away from the curb. It so easily tested my concentration and, for the longest time, plucked me out of the practice. Then one day, this teacher pointed out something that has stuck with me in many moments of everyday life: just because the bus goes by, it doesn't mean you have to get on.

With that thought came permission for me not to engage in "the static," all the noise around (and often within) that tended to pluck me out of present-time awareness. I could also let go of whatever thoughts proved unhealthy or irrelevant or were simply based on habits that did not serve me properly.

I believe sitting isn't the only way to meditate. I've actually found that some of my most awakened moments of meditation have been in the midst of a powerful *vinyasa* flow on my yoga mat. Likewise, there are times when I am chanting and a certain settling occurs, when everything becomes quite still and clear. In these moments I have moved from the effort of concentration into a place of noneffort. To me, this is the same state of meditation I aim for when sitting still. It is the space between thoughts.

There is no one correct technique for meditating; like the rest of yoga, take what works for you and leave what does not. For me, meditation is the art of listening. Sometimes I simply cannot do this for myself, so I think about someone dear to me who sometimes needs me to listen. To really hear what he or she is saying. To stop spacing out or pretending that I'm listening. To stop finishing their sentences or interrupting them. Sometimes my meditation becomes my exercise for being fully present in a moment that will never come again. I do not take this for granted. Everything we have, everyone we love, is on loan to us for just a short amount of time. We cannot go back in time and retrieve these moments.

I firmly believe that when we become completely present in any action in which we are engaged, we have set the stage for spontaneous meditation to occur. Even walking down the street is an opportunity to experience such present-time awareness.

Observe, focus, and then allow. Maybe you, too, will let the bus go by—especially if you really didn't need to get on in the first place.

A Note on Prayer versus Meditation

If you are anything like I was, you may be wondering what differentiates meditation from prayer. Prayer forms a major part of all religious practices today. Even among Hindus and Buddhists, there are likely more people praying than meditating. Prayer tends to be more easily understood, whereas meditation is more time-consuming and more challenging, and it requires serious and focused preparation.

I'd heard about meditation when I was growing up, but I had no idea how it differed from prayer. They seemed the same to me—except for the fact that the clergy from my church made it clear that I should avoid meditation. It fell into the same mystical realm as reincarnation and all things semi-taboo. I was taught that if I was sitting still in quiet repose, it should be in a moment of prayer. It has been a special journey discovering the difference between prayer and meditation.

My understanding of the distinction came when I allowed my inner voice to become quieter, when I began to take some control of my wandering mind. Prior to that, I didn't realize that there must be a moment to truly listen. To be so quiet, away from all the noise of the mind's chatter; to find that simple space where everything becomes clear and remarkably reassuring. As I learned to do this, moments arose when there was no disruption, not even a need to push away thoughts. It was here that I began to understand that meditation offers a glimpse into a stillness and union I had never known and that this practice was not in opposition to prayer, but rather a complement to it.

Interestingly, since understanding this, my prayers have become abundant with gratitude. I have found that counting and acknowledging my blessings allows me to be content in my life. I've also found that this has helped me to stop asking for all that much. I pray for the well-being of my family, friends, and community. I pray for healing. I have even begun to really understand the phrase "Thy will be done." In Sanskrit, there is a corresponding phrase that addresses how the Self and ultimate reality are not separate things: *tat tvam asi*, which translates to "that thou art."

This helps me immensely. I no longer need to try and beg or bargain for the impossible. If some calamity beyond my control happens despite my intervention and hopes, I have learned to pray more for acceptance than for anything that truly isn't in accord with life's natural course.

Thoughts on Beginning a Basic Seated Meditation

One of the best things about beginning a meditation practice is that there really isn't that much to do to prepare. Ultimately, this is a practice that can go with you just about anywhere and be tapped into at just about any time. But it will help to establish a basic foundation and routine in a comfortable place and at a convenient time.

If you have ever been on a long airline flight, you are familiar with all the hustle and bustle it takes to get you to the airport, through check-in and security, and finally into your seat. And then, what happens? You sit there. You sit there for hours. Maybe you will read or watch a movie. But think back to all the preparation that got you to this seat.

Getting ready to sit for meditation does not need to feel that complicated, but sometimes it can seem that way. There need not be anything frantic or complicated about this, though. I recommend that you allow it to be a sweet ritual without any worries or sense of shutting things out. When you prepare for meditation, you are setting out a welcome mat for your breath, mind, and heart. Please let it be easy and very positive. The only way it should be like the airport is in the taking off of your shoes.

SETTING UP

1. *Make time:* Choose a time of day that fits with your lifestyle. Although you can meditate at any hour, try and commit to a routine. Set a period of time for meditation that feels doable and will not be daunting. It doesn't have to be long. Even five minutes can be a great start.

2. *Set your environment:* Find a quiet place where there will be minimal to no distraction: no TVs, phones, and so on. Make certain the temperature is comfortable. If you wish, bring in scents or items you find beautiful or meaningful.

3. *Take a comfortable seat:* It may help to sit on a blanket or pillow. Many people like to have the cushion at a slightly downward angle, so their knees rest comfortably below their hips. This helps tilt the pelvis forward just a bit, allowing the vertebrae to stack properly. The main point of the seated position is to make sure your spine is straight. Make sure your arms and legs are relaxed. If sitting on the floor or on a cushion is uncomfortable, sit in a chair. Your hands can be cupped in your lap or resting on your thighs, however you are most comfortable.

4. *Scan your body:* Notice any parts of the body that are not relaxed and may be working unnecessarily. If there is tension in the back or face, make slight adjustments to find a better alignment. Relax the shoulders away from the ears.

TECHNIQUES TO TRY

Once you are set up and comfortable, try the following techniques. Use whichever one resonates with you. This may change from day to day, so check in each time you sit to see what feels right.

1. *Count your breaths:* Try watching your breath rise and fall. If possible, breathe only through your nose. Begin by exhaling completely, then inhale to the count of ten. At the top of the inhalation, take a slight pause. Then exhale to the count of ten. Continue. Make sure the length of each breath is comfortable. If counting to ten is too long or too short, chose a different count that feels right to you.

2. *Repeat a mantra:* If you have a sacred sound, repeat this silently or softly aloud.

3. *Concentrate on an object:* Chose something with *sattvic* (pure and balanced) qualities. *Sattvic* objects can include mantras (sacred sounds); *yantras* (sacred geometry); the breath; flowers; calligraphy of the symbol ом; images of deities, saints, or loved ones; or anything else you hold sacred. Begin by placing the object in front of you, then contemplate its positive qualities. Many people use the flame of a candle. Concentration happens when we intentionally push away thoughts unrelated to the object; meditation occurs when we sustain only thoughts related to the object.

For many of us, beginning to meditate is challenging. When we attempt to be still in the moment, when we do our best to pay attention, many internal and external forces try to battle for our attention. When this happens, smile. Be kind and compassionate, and notice how adorably human you really are. Then return to the exercise at hand.

At the same time, realize that you have already developed more concentration than you realize. If you've read this far, you've already demonstrated your ability to concentrate. Most of us know how to carry on a conversation while we are actually reading a book or paying attention to an interesting television program. Believe it or not, this could be the first step toward successful meditation!

Meditation may not be for everyone. If a seated meditation doesn't appeal to you, try practicing a moving meditation with your yoga practice. In Vinyasa Yoga, the meditation is on the movement of the body with the breath. This is another form of concentration practice.

Please know that you can be a happy and healthy person even if you never sit down and meditate. If you find that this is something that really doesn't suit you, be okay about it. But if you are someone whose mind runs nonstop all the time, this could very well be a great opportunity to befriend that meandering mind and help steer your thoughts in a healthier and more positive direction.

CHAPTER 5

The Yogic Diet

AYURVEDA, VEGETARIANISM, AND FOOD CHOICES THAT SUPPORT YOUR PRACTICE

THE PRACTICES OF BHAKTI YOGA and Bhakti Flow Yoga are lifestyle practices. When I was first introduced to the broader lifestyle of yoga, the practice took on a whole new meaning for me. In Bhakti Flow Yoga, we look at everything we can and see how to connect it all so we are living the life of which we dream. Many systems tend to celebrate only one part of the expansive tree of yoga, and while it is possible to study and "perfect" any single limb, leaf, or flower on this tree, I find it fascinating to try and understand all the parts as they relate to the whole. This is why the lifestyle of the practice is so important.

Many yoga practitioners come to the practice through the popular Hatha (physical) branch. But at some point, a lot of these students get restless and wonder not only what's next but, more profoundly, what they actually *do* with all these contortions. Sometimes this leads them to delve into the subtle energetic practices of breath awareness, meditation, or even the study of sacred texts.

Diet is a primary lifestyle choice that gets a lot of attention. It is natural to consider your diet once you have developed a routine with Hatha Yoga. We quickly learn that eating a full meal right before the physical practice makes it much more challenging and rather uncomfortable, so it's best to show up with an empty stomach along with an open mind and heart.

I notice that many students who understand the connection between food and exercise aim for diets that may be a bit extreme or, at the least, restrictive. You don't need a diet akin to self-torture to gain more flexibility, a theory that seems to be a trend in certain systems.

It is true that the food we ingest is our medicine. This nutrition is an essential aspect of our quality of life. It fuels this machine of a body. But we are each unique, and the fuel we need may not be the same as what someone else requires. For example, I live in a city with spectacularly gifted raw food chefs. The times I have adopted a raw foods diet, I did so with guidance, knowledge, and care. It was not casual. Yet even with that, I maintained a sense of hunger—and not necessarily a physical hunger. For me, it was a hunger for something warm and comforting. I sat with this a lot and tried to study it, move through it, even ignore it. Eventually, I realized that my very nature was asking for something different. To ignore this (literal and figurative) gut reaction was to miss the lesson at my (again, literal and figurative) core. So I have learned to weave a raw foods diet into my life when the time is right. Sometimes it is as simple as being seasonal, and other times it may be when I want to experience a cleansing.

In Bhakti Flow Yoga, we consider the whole practitioner: emotions, physical body, energetic body, and heart. The ancient Hindu system of medicine that is Ayurveda, meaning "knowledge of life," does much the same thing. Born of the knowledge of universal oneness, Ayurveda is likely the oldest life science known to civilization. Like the science of yoga, it originated in India's Vedic tradition thousands of years ago. Both of these complementary sciences came from the wisdom of those who had directly experienced the divine truth.

What follows is a brief introduction to Ayurveda to shed some light on lifestyle choices and habits. Once you have this knowledge, you simply choose what you do or don't want to keep. How cool is that?

Ayurveda

Fundamentally a science of healing and nurturing, Ayurveda is a holistic approach to health care as well as to mental and spiritual development. As a system, it aims to bring us into balance by addressing our personal characteristics and relating them to our lifestyle, including diet and hygiene. Don't worry that it might strip away your unique fabulousness. Rather, it's a way to recognize some common traits in our lifestyle choices and see how, under proper guidance, we can adjust these tendencies to bring us to a greater state of equanimity.

Respect and care for the environment is a main part of an Ayurvedic practice. Humans are a part of nature, and living in harmony with the universe is integral to our physical, intellectual, emotional, and spiritual development. Our responsibilities are twofold—to ourselves and to the environment. It is on this premise that Ayurveda's holistic approach to healing has developed.

Ayurvedic principles derive from the fundamental concept that all matter is composed of five elements: earth, water, air, fire, and ether. The ancient seers realized that these elements are but different manifestations of *prana*, the divine force that pervades the universe and is present in each of us. When these elements exist in balance, we are physically, mentally, and emotionally stable, whereas an imbalance between the elements can lead to various disturbances.

We are each born with our own unique combination of these elements. The way in which they come together defines our constitutional predisposition. Through the course of our lives, we may need to work on stabilizing or balancing our *prakruti* (inborn constitution). Ayurveda seeks to find our perfect point of balance, which is different for everyone. The first step is to ascertain our *dosha* (constitutional type). Depending on how the five elements combine within us, our natural constitution can be one or a combination of three types—*vata*, *pitta*, or *kapha*. Each *dosha* has certain defining physical, intellectual, and emotional characteristics that derive from the interplay of our internal energies as well as from our interaction with the environment. In working toward establishing harmony among the elements within us, we heal and nurture ourselves and refine our relationship with nature.

Unlike modern medical science, this ancient system does not aim to heal by treating only the symptoms of a disease. Rather, it seeks to understand the individual as a whole, looking for signs of internal imbalance as a possible cause of mental or physical ailments. The process of healing is through the restoration of balance, both within the individual and between the individual and nature.

The Doshas

A *vata*-type constitution is one in which the elements of air and ether are dominant. People with a *vata dosha* tend to be thin, mentally and physically quick, creative, and changeable. The predominance of air and ether gives *vata*-type individuals plenty of mobility on the physical and mental planes, so there is often a need for grounding. Lifestyle and diet are good ways to calm and balance *vata* and to help stabilize the inclination for excessive movement.

Here are the characteristics of a *vata* constitution:

- *Location:* Primarily in the nervous system, as well as in the rapid communication between neurons, but also in the colon, bones, joints, brain, skin, and ears
- *Physical effects of imbalance:* Dry skin, joint pain, abdominal gas, constipation, and nerve problems
- *Mental effects of imbalance:* Confusion, stress, fear, and loss of memory
- *Influences that aggravate* vata: Dry, cold, breezy weather; cold food and drink; gas-inducing (and some raw) foods; lack of routine; and too much travel
- *Influences that calm* vata: Warm, moist weather; a quiet, secure environment; a daily routine; rest and meditation; and warm, slightly oily, and moist food

Fire and water dominate *pitta*-type constitutions. People with a *pitta dosha* tend to be of medium build, muscular, strong-willed, and energetic. They often have good digestion because of the predominance of *agni* (fire) in their constitutions. *Pitta* types need to put their abundant energy to constructive use, or it may result in mood swings, anger, and other behavioral issues.

Here are the characteristics of a *pitta* constitution:

- *Location:* Primarily in the stomach and small intestine, but also in the blood, liver, gall bladder, spleen, and perspiration glands
- *Physical effects of imbalance:* Ulcers, rash, fever, sore throat, inflammation, sunburn, and kidney problems (The liver connection often shows up in the skin and eyes.)
- *Mental effects of imbalance:* Short temper, jealousy, irritability, frequent mood changes, and discontent
- *Things that aggravate* pitta: Hot weather and humidity; hot and oily food; too much salt, caffeine, meat, and alcohol
- *Things that calm* pitta: Cold weather and cool, airy environments; opportunities for the positive use of creative energy; cooling foods, dairy, whole grains, plenty of salads, and fresh fruit

Finally, *kapha*-type constitutions are characterized by a predominance of water and earth. Individuals with a *kapha dosha* are likely to be naturally heavy and have large bones. They are usually blessed with strength and staying power. When balanced, *kapha* types tend to be grounded, calm, and faithful. *Kapha* imbalances can lead to acquisitiveness, obsessive attachment, and *tamas* (inertia). Learning to let go of long-held habits and attitudes, which over time can lead to toxic internal buildups, can be beneficial for this *dosha*.

Here are the characteristics of a *kapha* constitution:

- *Location:* Primarily in the chest, but also in the lungs, nose, throat, mouth, head, joints, stomach, and lymph
- *Physical effects of imbalance:* Weight gain, sinus congestion, colds, sinusitis, headaches, edema, and diabetes
- *Mental effects of imbalance:* Lethargy, depression, excessive greed, lust, and attachment.
- *Things that aggravate* kapha: A sedentary lifestyle; too much routine; oily, sweet, and cold food; excess fluid
- *Things that calm* kapha: Regular exercise; changes from normal routine, challenge; fresh vegetables and whole grains, warm and light food.

AMA

Ama (toxic waste) is one of the fundamental concepts in the Ayurvedic system of healing. According to this system, wastes accumulate in the body as a result of poor diet and unhealthy lifestyle, leading to faulty digestion and assimilation. The toxins we breathe in also frequently collect in our tissues. It is well known that a body laden with accumulated wastes cannot function well. Following an appropriate diet for our *dosha* will decrease *ama* in our system.

Gunas

According to Sankhya, one of the traditional Indian schools of philosophy, *prakruti*, the world of phenomena that consists of mind and matter, has three fundamental *gunas* (qualities): *tamas*, *rajas*, and *sattva*.

Tamas is a state of inertia, darkness, ignorance, and indifference. From the perspective of evolution, it is the lowest level. A nature that is predominantly *tamas*-oriented makes a person ignorant, sluggish, and insensitive.

Rajas represents a state of energy and activity. This energy may manifest as passion, both positive and negative. Motivation, ambition, greed, lust, hatred, and anger are all *rajas*-like attributes. *Rajas* can also distract the mind and make a person selfish and egocentric. But a predominance of *rajas* also spurs people on to action and success, as motivation is a *rajas*-like attribute. It is a necessary stage in evolution and represents a higher state than *tamas*.

Sattva is the highest of the three *gunas*. It is a state of balance and harmony. When *sattva* dominates, a person has more control, is not swayed by ego, and tends to be detached and calm. Such a person is generally unselfish and compassionate.

These three *gunas* occur in different combinations in each of us and in every material phenomenon. However, the blend is not stable; like everything in nature, it keeps changing. In Sankhya thought, our journey from the world of mind and matter to the realm of the spirit progresses from *tamas* to *rajas* to *sattva* and finally transcends all three *gunas* into the stage beyond *sattva*, where we become one with universal energy. The true nature of the Self is said to be independent of the *gunas*; when consciousness transcends the *gunas* and becomes one with *purusha* (divine force), the Self is liberated. The influences of the three *gunas* are an important consideration in Ayurveda.

Nutrition in Ayurveda

In the course of their contemplation, the seers of ancient India discovered the holistic nature of life and the concept of universality, or unity of being. Food and humans are both a part of nature, and we have a responsibility to respect and nurture food sources. Our relationship with food not only affects the way we exist in our personal lives; it is also integral to universal harmony. When we choose to eat and live naturally, in ways that respect the laws of nature, we help to maintain balance on our planet. Nutrition plays a central role in Ayurvedic healing.

The Upanishads refer to food as *brahman* (the divine truth of the universe). Food comes from the divine and is offered to the divine in us. As such, it is best when it is pure, natural, and fresh, produced in harmony with nature. Such food nurtures our bodies, minds, and spirit. Unhealthy, processed, or stale food disrupts the flow of elemental energy within us and upsets the planetary balance.

As the seers of the past realized, and as we are beginning to understand today, a proper diet is one of the indispensable pillars of a healthy and meaningful life. It is unlikely that anyone can remain fit for long on an unhealthy, artificial diet or that any disease can be cured if the patient continues to eat improperly. Food is meant to cleanse, heal, and nourish, giving us the stability and vitality to develop physically, intellectually, and spiritually.

Ayurveda classifies food according to the *gunas*. As you would expect, *sattvic* foods are fresh, natural, and vegetarian. They cleanse the body and have a calming effect on the mind. In the past, *sattvic* foods were the prescribed diet for sages and monks. Ayurvedic nutrition has a strong *sattvic* emphasis because this type of food is considered nourishing and safe for people of all *doshas*. Examples of *sattvic* food are ghee (clarified butter), fresh fruit and vegetables, whole grains, pure dairy products, easily digestible pulses (legumes), and pure honey.

Rajasic foods are those that generate heat and spur a person to action. They have a stimulating effect on the mind and body. In ancient India, the diet of kings, soldiers, and those who lived predominantly material lives was mostly *rajasic*. Ayurveda does not prohibit *rajasic* food but advises moderation. Heat-inducing foods such as onions, garlic, hot spices and peppers, coffee, and alcohol are classified as *rajasic*.

Tamasic foods produce *ama* and therefore are best avoided. They induce inertia by making the mind and body sluggish. Regular intake of *tamasic* food can make the body vulnerable to disease. Junk and processed food, meat, fish, cheese, and any food that is stale, has chemicals, is fried, or is excessively oily, spicy, or sweet is *tamasic* in nature. Alcohol is considered both *rajasic* and *tamasic*.

Taste and Its Role in Ayurvedic Nutrition and Healing

Understanding the concept of taste, or *rasa*, from an Ayurvedic perspective is vital to being able to nourish and heal ourselves. According to Ayurveda, the therapeutic properties of food derive from the effects of taste. Ayurveda defines six tastes and their impact on the body. Taste also influences mental and emotional states. For example, sweet taste in moderation can make us feel good and generate love and kindness, whereas too much of it can bring on *tamas*.

Balancing tastes according to our *dosha* is healing and nourishing. *Vata*-type constitutions, for example, respond well to the lubricating effect of moist tastes, which help to counter some of that constitution's inherent dryness.

Sweet taste is composed of the elements earth and water:

- *Gunas:* Heavy and moist
- *Immediate effect:* Cooling; can inhibit digestion to some extent
- *Long-term effect:* Can increase moisture and weight if eaten in large quantities
- Dosha *compatibility:* Good for *vata* and *pitta* in moderation; can aggravate *kapha*

Salty taste is composed of the elements fire and water:

- *Gunas:* Heavy and moist
- *Immediate effect:* Warming; stimulates digestion
- *Long-term effect:* Moistening; can cause water retention if consumed in excess
- Dosha *compatibility:* Benefits *vata*; not as good for *pitta* because of mild heat; beneficial for *kapha* because of warmth but not in its tendency to promote moisture retention and weight gain

Sour taste is composed of the elements earth and fire:

- *Gunas:* Slightly heavy and moist
- *Immediate effect:* Warming; good for digestion and warming for the system
- *Long-term effect:* Warming and moistening; can cause some fluid retention
- Dosha *compatibility:* Especially good for *vata* because it stimulates digestion and generates warmth and moisture; can aggravate *pitta* and *kapha* if consumed in excess

Pungent taste is composed of the elements fire and air:

- *Gunas:* Dry and light
- *Immediate effect:* Hot; stimulates digestion
- *Long-term effect:* Hot, light, and dry; has a warming effect and relieves excess humidity in the body
- Dosha *compatibility:* Particularly useful for *kapha*; good for *vata* in small quantities, but too much can have a dehydrating effect; tends to aggravate *pitta* and can be tolerated only if blended with other tastes

Astringent taste is composed of the elements earth and air:

- *Gunas:* Somewhat light and dry
- *Immediate effect:* Cooling; tends to slow digestion
- *Long-term effect:* Dry and light; can inhibit the circulation of blood and enzymes

- Dosha *compatibility:* Beneficial for *pitta* because it counteracts heat; helps balance *kapha* by neutralizing excess moisture and weight; aggravates *vata* by increasing dryness and cold

Bitter taste is composed of the elements ether and air:

- *Gunas:* Light and somewhat dry
- *Immediate effect:* Cooling (In India, a small amount of bitter vegetables is often eaten at the beginning of a meal to stimulate appetite.)
- *Long-term effect:* Light and dry
- Dosha *compatibility:* Good for *pitta*, particularly for digestion; can help pacify *kapha*; tends to upset *vata* and is best consumed in small quantities or in combination with other tastes

Ayurveda does not forbid the eating of meat and fish but considers them *tamasic.* Regular consumption of these proteins is known to increase *ama.* In the past, organic meat and fish produced by relatively nonviolent means were consumed for nourishment. However, animal protein is more difficult to digest than plant-based protein and is best consumed in moderation, if at all.

Vegetarian food, on the other hand, is easy to digest and assimilate, is nourishing to the body, and prevents the accumulation of toxic wastes. Also, it can be produced by nonharmful methods. Ayurveda, with its focus on maintaining harmony within ourselves and in nature, advocates a nonviolent approach to living. By harming another life, we upset the balance in nature and ultimately harm ourselves.

In Ayurveda, general health and digestive ability go together. Digestive ability is known as *agni.* Burping, poor appetite, constipation, gas, and acidity (specifically, acid reflux and indigestion) are all signs of poor digestive ability. One of the essentials of good digestion is a relatively *ama*-free system. The presence of toxic waste not only retards digestion but is also the source of many diseases. Eating the right kind of food in appropriate combinations and amounts helps prevent the accumulation of *ama* in the body. Hot foods and spices stimulate digestion, whereas cold foods tend to slow it down. This is why Ayurveda recommends eating a combination of hot and cold foods.

A diet comprising tastes useful for our *dosha* heals and nourishes over the short and long term. It is also important to balance tastes according to the seasons; for example, cooling foods are helpful in summer, whereas warming, heavy foods are comforting in winter.

Ayurvedic Nutritional Guidelines for Good Digestion and General Health

The recommendations for a healthy diet offered by ancient texts, such as the Charaka Samhita, are relevant even today. Here are a few of them:

- It is best not to eat more than one type of concentrated protein at a time.
- Food is most easily digestible, safe, and nourishing when cooked and warm.
- Food is best eaten on an empty stomach.
- Tasty food stimulates and aids digestion.
- Food needs to be consumed in appropriate quantities. Overeating or eating too little are both bad for digestion.
- Eat foods that are suited to your *dosha* and general health.
- Eat in a calm, pleasant environment.
- Relax at mealtimes and be aware of what you are eating.
- Rushing through a meal or lingering too long are not digestion-friendly approaches.

The Vegetarian Emphasis

I have chosen to be vegetarian and vegan most of my life. I first adopted this diet out of rebellion: I come from a family of hunters and fishermen, but I could never make sense of the sport of killing an animal. Later, being vegetarian was all about getting as healthy as I could. There was another point when I came to really understand how eating "low on the food chain" was much less harmful to the planet. Then I found a more philosophical reason to remain on this path. And now, when I am asked why I am vegetarian, I simple say, "All of the above."

To me, the practice of Bhakti Yoga is a complete lifestyle. It is about honoring all beings. This includes the two-legged, four-legged, finned, winged, and feathered. Human beings have the opportunity to be caretakers of the planet. The idea that any of these beings are food doesn't make sense to me.

It is an ancient yogic principle that the food we ingest affects not only our body but also our mind. A Sanskrit saying that best reflects the belief that lies at the root of India's long experience with vegetarianism is *Ahimsa paramo dharma*, meaning "Nonviolence is the highest dharma." *Prana* is not just the vital force that gives us life; it also lets animals breathe. Killing an animal involves robbing it of *prana* and disturbing the flow of this universal force, thereby also doing harm to those who do the killing. Respect and love for all beings is one of the underlying concepts of yoga; great yogis have always emphasized that an animal's right to live is as fundamental as a human's.

When I began practicing a certain style of yoga many years ago, I was immediately attracted to the system's insistence on students being vegetarian. But then I sensed that this insistence was closer to being dogma. I wondered if students of this school became vegetarian only because it was required. If so, how could that be sustained? And might it not backfire later if a student became resentful of being "forced" into this part of the yoga lifestyle?

This reminds me of the shock tactics some animal rights advocates use to encourage vegetarianism. I think it is vital that we know where our food comes from, and it is wise to see this process as close to firsthand as possible. But to share this information in a violent manner seems unwise, unkind, and counterproductive. I think we can educate in a compassionate manner rather than trying to shock someone into reality. When the messenger is so severe, the message itself can be lost or dismissed.

In my early days of vegetarianism, I fell for this impractical approach and was loud, insistent, and completely obnoxious. When I ceased this behavior, I was amazed at how many people would come to me of their own volition and ask that I share my story and how they, too, might begin this path.

With this experience in mind, my intention here is to inform and invite, not to insist or require anything at all. If and when the time is right for you to give it a try, consider adopting a plant-based diet for a short time, just to see how it fits into your lifestyle. But do this with mindfulness and respect. Keep your plate filled with colorful, nutritious, and delicious foods. Be creative and think about what you are adding to your diet, not about what you are taking away. This awareness will make your exploration much more successful.

The term *vegetarian* was coined in the 1840s, when the Vegetarian Society of the United Kingdom was founded. Since then, the term has come to include different eating patterns, not all of which restrict themselves to plant-based foods alone. The notion that vegetarian diets are not as strengthening as meat-based diets is a misconception. Quite a few world-class athletes are vegetarian, and it's becoming easier to find recipes and instructions for how to be a high-performance athlete on a vegetarian or vegan diet. Indeed, the understanding that being totally or partially vegetarian is a sensible and ethical choice is gaining wider acceptance in many countries.

Here are some vegetarian dietary choices to consider if you are interested:

- A *vegan* diet excludes all animal-based products, including dairy and eggs. Some vegans even avoid honey, gelatin, and marshmallows.
- A *lacto-vegetarian* diet includes dairy products but excludes all other animal foods.
- An *ovo-vegetarian* diet includes eggs but excludes dairy and other animal foods.
- A *lacto-ovo-vegetarian* diet includes dairy products and eggs but not meat, fish, chicken, or other flesh.

The reassuring message that both yoga and Ayurveda have for humanity is that we can transform our lives for the better if we will. I have seen this transformation in my own life and in the lives of many others. Food is our nutrition, and our diet reflects our care for this bodily vessel and the planet we inhabit. My own plant-based diet gives me all the nutrients I need and the assurance that the practice of *ahimsa* (nonharming) is my contribution to a better life and more compassionate care of the environment.

CHAPTER 6

On Teaching

If you find a job you really love, you'll never work again.
— WINSTON CHURCHILL

LIKE MANY INSTRUCTORS, I came to teaching as a natural extension of my own practice. Teaching yoga often becomes part of the evolution of the practice, although you *always* remain a student. The teacher— or teacher-to-be—who has been profoundly touched by the positive effects of yoga on any level can draw from that grace-filled experience and offer a voice that is genuine and luminous. It is from that enthusiasm that passion emerges and knowledge is shared. Having full faith in what you are teaching truly matters. My experiences led me to the development of Bhakti Flow Yoga, and it is through these experiences that I developed these teaching tools. However, it does not matter what form of yoga you teach or want to teach; the tools remain the same.

I remember once speaking with a dedicated student who really wanted to become a teacher but shyly admitted that he couldn't teach because he was unable to touch his own toes. I thought, *How wonderful!* This person knows about the effort involved but is simply stymied by some irrelevant destination. This is the making of the special kind of teacher to whom I am attracted and the kind of teacher I strive to be: one who is still evolving and can speak humbly yet passionately about the journey itself. I am far more inspired by the journey involved in trying to touch one's toes than by the actual ability to do so.

That's why the practice of yoga isn't necessarily a system for improving the self; it's much more about self-acceptance. In fact, as teachers, just about the most compassionate thing we can do is to remind students that they are okay as they are. Something in our society has convinced every one of us that we are lacking or that we dare not live our dreams or allow ourselves to open to the qualities we truly admire in others. Yet these qualities are already within us. Yoga practice can help awaken that awareness and permit us to realize that potential. We already have everything we need.

I never planned on teaching as much as I have, and I certainly never anticipated that I would get to share this beautiful practice with the many students I have been so blessed to serve. Along the way, I have "checked" myself by maintaining a deep gratitude and respect for the impermanence of the experience. Amazingly, the notion of yogic nonattachment has proved to be the most rewarding by-product of this approach to teaching. I remind myself not to cling, because nothing is permanent—not asanas, not studios, not students, not even teachers.

In this chapter, I offer a few thoughts to inspire your own personal creativity and joy for the practice. Please remember these are just my opinions, and they are subject to change as I continue to evolve on my own path. There are exceptions to everything written here. I hope you will try out all the options and see what is right for you. I hear some teachers say "never" do this and "never" do that. I spent the early part of my existence being told "never." I'm going to spend my remaining days thinking, *Maybe. Just maybe.*

My Path to Teaching

I remember the first teacher with whom I studied. What a lasting impact! My initiation into the practice was with someone stern but effective; he was grumpy and kind of mean. At the time, I thought this was how it was supposed to be. I still loved him, of course, because he helped me get to know myself and helped me reconnect my body and mind in ways I'd long forgotten.

When I began teaching, I wanted to be effective too, but I knew that being kind and supportive could generate an equal, if not better, result than being stern. So I began my quest to become a teacher who could instruct with grace, kindness, and a genuine belief that students have an inner reservoir of energy, a reservoir that may have only rarely been tapped. I wanted to be a cheering instructor who could help bring that out.

I hadn't been in search of a new career when I took my first training, and I wasn't trying to earn extra income. I was already working a full-time job in an acute health care setting. In addition, I worked on-call much of the time and spent most of my remaining hours either on my yoga mat or fast asleep. I took my first yoga teacher training program simply to delve deeper into my own practice. But when a studio owner asked if I would start teaching a class on Fridays at 6 A.M., I realized this was one of the few spaces in my schedule when I could actually give it a try. It was exhilarating and quickly became my favorite time of the week.

I believe two main factors led me to embrace the art of teaching, and they are the qualities I feel have most enhanced my success and longevity as a teacher. First was my love for the practice. Being on the mat has, since the beginning, meant so much to me, and watching myself transform on so many levels continues to impact me deeply. It was and remains the most natural shift into loving self-awareness I have ever known. My heart had never danced so freely, and every cell in my body felt alive.

From that great enthusiasm was born my voice, the second of the qualities I believe are necessary to be a teacher. I wanted to share the practice with everyone. I just couldn't shut up about it. My office at the hospital became a small sanctuary, with warm lighting, along with photos and posters relating to yoga on my shelves and walls. My mat sat rolled and ready in the corner.

I found that I could speak clearly about my experience. Sharing the journey was easy, and I couldn't help but notice how contagious that joyful energy could be. If you possess passion for the practice and can talk about it in an informed and articulate way, you have just about everything you need to be successful.

Although our experiences are unique historically and culturally, it is important to make sure that we always remain students of the teachings that have come before us. I would like to emphasize how important continuing education is. A teacher should have a teacher. A teacher is always a student. A student is always a beginner. A beginner should always be willing to say, "I don't know." Surrender to a state of constant inquiry.

Continually absorbing the teachings of our ancestors is just one approach to furthering our studies. I believe it is also important to develop empathy by interacting with others in our day-to-day lives. Our healthy conduct in all relationships is a key to great awakening and awareness. Really listening to others will help all our relationships grow stronger and more heartfelt. My friend Will, in almost every conversation with just about anyone, says, "You're absolutely right," even when I know he doesn't actually agree. It always cracks me up, but on some level, what I hear him saying is, "Your truth is just as important to you as my truth is to me, so there is no need to argue about anything." Can you imagine a world where we let everyone's voice be heard and didn't feel an incessant need to criticize, argue with, or belittle what they have to say? What if, instead, we listened and considered carefully how they have come to their view and allow it to be as it is?

My everyday observances help make me a better teacher. I watch a mom at the grocery store juggling babies and coupons and an amazingly full life, and I can't help but wonder why I can't do better at keeping my own act together day to day. She becomes a teacher to me, showing me balance, flexibility, and strength. I remember her when I go to my mat, and she helps me stay in Chair Pose (Utkatasana) a bit longer or find balance and grace in Lord of the Dance Pose (Natarajasana). I then dedicate my practice to her. I believe that my practice can somehow find her out there in the world and bring her comfort and consolation.

As I teach, I look for her in the room. Well, maybe not *her*, but someone who might have similar struggles. It could be a parent, sibling, child, partner, or sweetheart: I know that he or she is here looking for guidance, balance, strength, empowerment, and possibly even refuge. My noticing that person in everyday life helps me to recognize him or her in the yoga room.

I have also been greatly inspired by the simple practices recommended by Swami Sivananda and Swami Vishnudevananda: selfless service to remove egoism, mantra chanting and worship to release emotion into devotion and selfless love, study of the scriptures to transcend the intellect, and meditation to go deeply within and arrive at the true nature of our being. Much of this has helped me in creating my own expression of the practice.

Being a Teacher

Having a clear understanding of why we are teaching and what it is we want out of the experience can help us stay connected to the lifelong journey of learning, unfolding, and sharing the secret that exists well below the surface. If we are here to serve, whom or what do we aim to serve? Being clear about that direction of energy and intention and recognizing our place in it makes a big difference.

I want to find service in the heart of the Beloved. I want to serve those in need. But in the past, I have shortchanged my ability to serve by not taking care of myself properly. To be of service, we first need to make sure we are okay. I liken this to preparing for a journey—making sure I am fit and packed and have my compass and map ready. To be haphazard about my well-being doesn't do justice to my ultimate opportunity to make an impact. As with the physical yoga practice, what we put in determines what we get out.

Empathy is one of the most important attributes a teacher can develop. To experience a sense of similarity while recognizing another person's differences helps us to see who is actually in front of us and not just who we think he or she should be. Other people's life experiences are obviously quite different from ours. Yet there is, unquestionably, a common thread between us all. Being present and clear can help us see that common thread. It is not an easy task to set aside all of our own preconceptions and prejudices. But if we are teachers who are really here to serve, what greater gift can we offer the blessed beings who have found their way into our care than present-mind awareness? My aim is to be fully present in each experience so I can serve to the best of my ability.

One challenge in developing empathy is being careful not to project what we are feeling (or what we have felt in the past) onto others. My life experiences will not be the same as yours. My joys and losses cannot possibly be the same as yours. Certainly my hamstrings, hips, and shoulder blades cannot be the same as yours. But through intuitive inquiry, observation, and listening, we can understand more about where others have been and what it is they may be seeking. For example, when a friend of mine lost her mother, I knew that although I experienced the heartbreak of losing my own mother, I still didn't know what it was like to lose hers. I created space for her to tell me. To practice understanding others, we must listen on every level. For teachers who remain trapped in a monologue, this may prove to be a real test.

We are here to serve with open and compassionate hearts. We are lifeguards entrusted to look after those in our care, to make sure they are safe and supported. It is an amazing opportunity to help create this refuge.

In the course of practice and teaching, I have been able to change my mind often. The truths we hold now should be open to reevaluation and remain in sync with the evolution of our personal path. Evolving as a student is essential for keeping the practice alive, both for our own well-being and for the development and interests of the students we serve. Continuing education and personal exploration are integral to that expansion of consciousness.

When I am teaching, I share the ideals that I personally strive toward on and off the mat. I have learned that each time we stand in the room as teachers and leaders, we have choices. We can choose courage and lead from a heart filled with loving-kindness, or we can choose fear and lead with arrogance and superiority. I've tried both, and I firmly believe that the artful discipline of yoga must be instilled in a loving, nurturing, and supportive manner, one that invites an atmosphere of self-discovery and creative expression. There is a way to encourage students toward great empowerment, acceptance, and balance without pushing them. There is a way to encourage introspection without the need for self-deprecation or self-absorption. It is important to recognize the difference.

However creative we may long to be as teachers, it is important that we teach only what we know. Our words should reflect our own experiences. For example, I teach only the asanas I understand. If something doesn't feel right to me, I set it on the back burner. I do not expound on philosophies I know little about. I do not teach dogma, because I've had enough of that in my life. I share the tools I have found to be healthful, transformational, and liberating.

The language we use is important as well. Be clear and direct with your speech. Sometimes, instructing in different ways can help facilitate a better understanding for everyone in the room. If you say something once and students do not respond, repeating the same words in the same tone (or getting snappy) only brings more confusion. Take on this challenge with great enthusiasm. It is a lesson in empathy. Try to remember that students *want* to do what you are asking of them. They just might not understand you. Help them with kindness.

I try not to use the phrases "my students," "my teacher," or "my classes." None of these belongs to me. Be aware of language and how your choice of words relates to your attachment to any current experience in your life. For me, the students are "students we are blessed to serve." The teacher becomes "the teacher from whom I draw inspiration." The classes are "the classes I am blessed to lead."

I know that many of the people I work with are looking for a creative and effective workout. While the classes I lead tend to be vigorous and physically challenging, their actual power stems from each student's internal experience. When I first started teaching, the experience was softer. The atmosphere was quiet and sweet because I thought folks just needed to come to a serene sanctuary. But I began to notice that many people still fidgeted like crazy and fought against the quiet, even though it seemed like there was a craving for it. I realized that those of us who are urban dwellers and surrounded by stimulation might need our yoga experience to reflect that intensity so we could settle down from it. I decided to take it up a notch or so. The intensity, the heat, the music—everything became more powerful and alive.

As the classes grew stronger, I knew to keep looking for those places in the "chaos" when everything would suddenly connect and flow so sweetly together so that it afforded the most magical of moments, almost as if all the windows and doors were gently opened. This is when I offer a pearl of yogic wisdom, perhaps a bit about what this dear practice means to me. In the softest of those splendid teaching moments, it's almost like the unraveling of a quilt that has taken a lifetime to sew. People are sometimes scared to let go of what they've spent their lives thinking is right or wrong. My goal is to let students know that they are so very powerful and so much more okay than they may realize. Since for me this practice is about self-acceptance rather than self-improvement, it is important to make clear that whatever shifts are happening in the practice are already part of the individual. A powerful *vinyasa* practice can shake things up to the point of calming things down. This is when many of us allow a pure sense of "okayness" to pervade. This is the essence of *santosha* (contentment). It brings to mind those quiet moments after a storm, when everything becomes still.

Students will come to you with great trust. Remember that we are in the service industry. We are here to serve, not to be served. Some students will want to put you on a pedestal. Allowing this to happen will inevitably bring suffering to you both. Falling (or being pushed) from that pedestal is almost inevitable. You may also find that some students will want more from you than you can afford to give. Be comfortable establishing boundaries. Find the healthy balance of being kind and supportive without becoming involved in students' personal lives or decision-making processes. You can be friendly without being friends. If you are the teacher, be the teacher. I have boundaries, such as not accepting social invitations from students. It's important that you learn what your own boundaries are and be willing to communicate them clearly in your actions and words. But remember, having boundaries is not the same thing as creating a wall between yourself and the beings in your care. Such an obstacle does not serve the role of teacher.

Sometimes students want you to be a counselor or adviser, or they simply want you to know things you don't. Direct them to a health care provider, counselor, mechanic, accountant, or whomever they need. In many cases, the three most important words a teacher should be comfortable saying are "I don't know." Remaining a beginner secures the essential qualities of humility and respect in the relationship between student and teacher. From that type of relationship comes the opportunity for students to witness the teacher's rawness and flaws. This is important, a gift the teacher gives the students. From there, if the students are projecting anything else, the teacher can offer it back to them.

Of course, as yoga teachers, there are many reasons why we sometimes don't feel like inspiring the masses, being a cheerleader, or being profound. There are days when we have our own stuff going on, or we just don't feel well physically, mentally, or emotionally. Sometimes we are not well rested. Other times we may feel insecure and even incompetent. And there are times when we would much rather curl up alone and not even be there. We are human.

But it is important for us to remember that we are here to be of service, and that service should never be affected by whatever fleeting moments of fatigue, doubt, insecurity, or off-centeredness we may feel. In these moments, I remind teachers to fulfill their duty, sometimes setting aside their personal stuff, and remember that those coming to practice with us need us to offer the work we signed up for. We really do have only a short "shift" and can certainly stay focused on our essential role of serving others for that hour and a half.

A few practical reminders: Be clean, showered, and well kempt before teaching—no body odors or colognes/perfumes. Make sure your hands and feet are clean and your nails are trimmed. Be aware of any jewelry you may wear; for instance, loud bracelets can be a distraction and can also interfere with assisting students. If you are sick or feel like you may be catching something, don't touch anyone. The practice of *ahimsa* means that we take care of ourselves so we can take care of others. Take time off when you need to. And if a student has personal effects such as glasses or jewelry that he or she puts next to the mat, consider placing these items on top of a block so you do not accidentally step on them while walking around or adjusting.

Remember, yoga is for everyone, not just the young and fit. Let yourself share this practice with everyone who may be interested. I feel blessed to teach people of all shapes and sizes. I've worked with people who can't get down to the floor. I've taught chair yoga to senior citizens aged eighty-two to ninety-six. When I am with students, I'm in love, filled with appreciation for how powerful they are and how hard they try. I am in constant awe, inspired by people offering everything they have in each moment.

Most of all, as teachers and students, when we believe in the practice and what it has to offer, everything else flows. A student recently asked me a simple question: "Why do we do yoga?" Out of the many reasons that came to mind, this answer came before all the others and I knew that it was the right one: "Many of us come to yoga because something or someone in our lives once told us we weren't good enough or something is wrong with us, and we've yet to make peace with that or find out how completely untrue it really is. The practice, much like a good friend, finds us at just the right time and blesses us with the understanding that we are more connected and more okay than we assumed we were."

Thus, we as teachers have a uniquely profound opportunity to share this message of light with those who have lived in the darkness for long enough.

PART TWO

The Poses

CHAPTER 7

Introduction to the Poses

Consider this body to be on loan. In fact, consider everything we have—our senses, talents, intellect, relationships, and experiences—to be on loan. We certainly don't know how long they will be in our possession, but we do know there is some type of expiration date.

If we could stop the clock somehow and take a look at where we have been and where we (think we) are going, wouldn't we make more conscious decisions about how we use whatever time we have left? In yoga, we can appreciate that we have been offered only a certain number of breaths in this existence. If we knew how many we had left, we most likely would use them with much greater care and awareness. This is a perfect way to honor the practice. The breath is what keeps us here. It is what helps us thrive and communicate. Paying attention to the breath is what grounds us in this moment. Wisdom tells us that once we have found appreciation for where we are right now, it is important to look at where we have been and how that defines who we are. From this perspective, we can carefully decide where we would like to go from here.

To delve into that awareness completely, the practice of Hatha Yoga gives us the opportunity of using our physical body to explore our immediate and past history and its impact on who we really are. This exploration of mind through the body and the breath is a journey of compassionate self-discovery. There is no self-deprecation and nothing harsh about this process. It is a journey of love and great kindness. It begins from deep within so that it can ultimately move with humble authenticity beyond the self; thus, it is important to keep the mind clear and present as we look within. In this practice, we stretch, twist, churn, contort, strengthen, balance, and yoke the body in ways that are often beyond our imagination at the beginning. And that is when everything becomes interesting.

Observing our thought patterns ultimately helps steer the direction of our yoga practice. Within every asana, we are contending with our mental workings. It is the mind itself that creates the poses of the body. In even the simplest yoga poses, we learn a lot about our avoidances and attachments. An obvious example is when a teacher calls out a pose we really don't want to do. In that moment, most of us have already decided what we are going to put into it, if anything at all. Another example is how excited we are when coming into a pose we really like or in which we know we look good. It is also easy to notice any self-imposed limitations. With a readily available sense of awareness, this is a great place to play with the attitudes that seem to define us, even a little.

Recognizing these reactions, as well as noticing what we normally put into the experience—and then being willing to change something even slightly—alters our entire habit of thought and thus the yoga pose itself. We have then learned to confront head-on a thought pattern that may have been with us for a long time. We become familiar with the sense of empowerment, excitement, and even liberation in those precious moments. We have learned to change our minds, exhibiting the most powerful form of flexibility.

> We gain strength and courage and confidence by each experience in which we really stop to look fear in the face. . . . We must do that which we think we cannot.
>
> — ELEANOR ROOSEVELT

It is said that a pose truly begins the moment you want to leave it. Many yoga poses are meant to challenge on all levels: physically, emotionally, and mentally. Notice what happens in the moment when you want to exit the pose. Is your mind telling you it is time to run when you start to feel a little uncomfortable? When you choose to stay in the pose, that is often when things start to happen. When you persevere through the physical and mental challenge, when you choose to stay with it, you can feel yourself getting stronger and less reactive and finding a place of equanimity. It is like life. It gets harder, and then it gets easier, so try and breathe past your initial discomfort to see what is on the other side. In fact, look for that space between comfort and discomfort.

Everything about who we are in our lives is revealed to us through these poses. Allow yourself to listen to and look carefully at whatever it is you are feeling. Be compassionate in this state. Be kind as you observe patterns that may come up. Are you someone who runs when things get difficult or a bit scary? Or are you someone who draws on your own inner strength and goes into situations knowing that you have the tools you need to move through rough times with grace? Behind the heart, there is courage. Behind the heart, there is also fear. We are blessed to be able to choose one or the other at any given time.

Drishti Matters

Drishti refers to the soft-gazing point we use in the practice. This technique, along with Ujjayi Pranayama (Victorious Breath), *bandhas* (energetic locks that help regulate energy), and the dedication of the practice, help create the stage where spontaneous meditation can be born.

The practice of *drishti* is both powerful and enlightening, but it is not at all easy. There are so many visual distractions throughout the day that it is easy to get lost in those distractions, even in the yoga room. We tend to look around and check everything out. But when we do that, what exactly happens? Once we start scoping out the yoga room, whether intentionally or unwittingly, most of us can easily slip into judging everything and everyone we see. A focused gaze can remedy that. It can also give us the opportunity to be more present in the moment and in the experience of the asana.

I notice that when students look around the room, they get concerned about what their neighbors are doing. Think about it. If your neighbor gets up in the middle of class and your eyes follow him out of the room, isn't your mind going with him? The next thing you know, you might start thinking that maybe you need to go too. Now and again, I ask students to go ahead, look around the room, and check everything out. Notice everyone and what they are wearing and just get it out of the way. Then I ask them to come back to the real exercise at hand: to steady the mind and be in this moment, a moment that will never come again.

Even in a home practice, it's easy to get distracted. Try not to get caught up visually by your surroundings. The key is to notice what is there but try not to create any stories about it. Allow whatever it is to be fine as it is— no avoidance and no attachment.

A set *drishti* helps us get through challenging poses. Instead of searching for a distraction to help us "survive" the moment, we have the opportunity to tune right in to the experience and learn something about ourselves, such as how we get attached to certain sensations or how we run away from them.

Some systems of yoga encourage specific *drishti* points. I suggest certain directions for your gaze, but I always point out that if it isn't comfortable, change it. If looking straight up feels reasonable, do that. If looking forward or down is better, honor that. It's all about *ahimsa*, that space of nonharming.

It's also important to let *drishti* have a journey. For example, instead of looking at one spot on the ceiling in a standing backbend, consider using the *drishti* to draw a line with your eyes from the floor in front of you up the wall and then to the ceiling and beyond, if appropriate. Even in Warrior II Pose (Virabhadrasana), I ask students to consider not just staring beyond their fingers, but to notice their entire arm and hand along the way. This isn't about getting caught up in the object you're gazing at;

it is really about taking advantage of even that moment of observation to learn just a bit more about ourselves.

There is an inner *drishti* too, that gazing point inside each of us. Perhaps it is like an inner compass that helps us find our way in daily life, especially in the midst of suffering and calamities. Sometimes to discover that inner *drishti*, we need to set up an environment in which it can make itself known. Many of the techniques and tools presented in the following chapters give us that quiet, clear place where both inner and outer vision can emerge.

Some Thoughts on Setting Up a Practice

Create time in your day for a regular practice, and aim for the same time each day, if possible. At first, you may want to try practicing at different times and see what works best for your lifestyle and disposition. For many of us, a morning practice is best because the mind is easier to focus; however, the body may be a bit tighter and more resistant. You may find your body to be much more open in the afternoon or early evening, but the trade-off could be that your mind is a bit busier. Try and commit to at least one hour per day and up to 90 minutes, if possible. If this isn't realistic for your lifestyle, don't worry! Try 30 to 45 minutes and see if that fits your schedule. Offer what you can afford.

Consider a place in your home that has the necessary space, cleanliness, warmth, calm, and privacy for your practice. If you have to move furniture every time you put your mat down, you may be less inclined to develop a regular routine. It doesn't take much space, so look around and see what works for you. Let this become your sacred space. Bless it however you like. Candles, incense, photos of loved ones and deities, music that inspires you, and whatever else brings you inner peace and positive influences can help make this practice space your special refuge. Your yoga mat will become your magic carpet. Even when I travel, I create this space everywhere I stay.

Use the poses that follow as a launching pad for your practice. In the pose directions, look for the modifications section for opportunities to go deeper or ease up within the pose. Play with those to find the ones that work best for you in each moment. Begin with some of the basic poses and then start having fun. Consider what your body wants to do each day rather than imposing something else on it.

A good way to put together a well-rounded practice is to choose a few poses from each of these chapters that follow. Try this order: standing poses, arm balances, inversions, backbends, twists, forward bends, and finally, restorative poses. I like to sprinkle core work throughout my practice to maintain my awareness of these key muscles in many of the poses, but you can put core work wherever you like. Experiment and see what feels good to you. If you'd like to start with something ready-made, I have included a sequence that I call Surya Flow at the end of this book. It's a one-hour class outline I designed for early morning practitioners.

The relaxation at the end of the practice is a very important element. It helps to integrate all the work from the other poses. The world is a safer place when you give yourself permission to relax.

If you choose to attend a class, make sure to attend one at the most appropriate level for you. Many people make the mistake of starting with a class that is too difficult, especially if they have an athletic background. They think they can escape the fundamentals. Trust that you can build the fundamentals quickly, but if you don't start with them, it's hard to go back and unlearn what you've done incorrectly, especially with breathing. Also realize that yoga offers a noncompetitive environment. If you are a competitive person, do your best to set that aside with yourself and others during practice. The advice I give to both beginners and seasoned practitioners is that there is no room for ambition or greed in yoga. Neither will serve you, and both can be ineffective or detrimental.

If you are pregnant, or if you have a history of high or low blood pressure, refer to the guidelines at the end of this book. And, as with any new exercise routine, be sure to consult with your health care provider before you begin.

CHAPTER 8

Basics

FOUNDATIONAL POSES help ground us and should never be underestimated. They may seem relatively simple, but the truth is you can easily spend an entire lifetime studying each and every one. Allow them to help with positive mind training; as you develop concentration and focus in these poses, you will find more confidence in your abilities on and off the mat. Let your work in these poses become your passion, and let the poses themselves provide a safe haven for returning to the roots of your practice.

DOWNWARD-FACING DOG POSE (ADHO MUKHA SVANASANA)

Getting In

- Start on your hands and knees in Table Pose (Bharmanasana). Align your knees under your hips and your hands under and slightly in front of your shoulders, fingers pointed forward. Curl your toes under.
- Inhale and drop your belly toward the floor as you lift your tailbone in Cow Pose (Bitilasana), creating a shallow bowl shape with your spine.
- As you exhale, raise your hips by pressing into your hands and feet while straightening your legs and arms until they are fully extended.
- Your feet should be hip-width apart, with the outside edges of your feet parallel to the edges of your mat.
- In the full pose, your torso, neck, and arms are on one straight plane, and your neck is elongated. Do not let your neck or head fall below your arms.

- Feel your shoulder blades broaden across your back as your arms lengthen, moving your shoulders away from your ears.
- Contract your thighs.
- To deepen the stretch, lift your hips and sit bones and lengthen your spine. Gently press your heels toward the earth.
- Gaze toward your navel or between your calves.
- Breathe deeply. Hold for 5 to 10 breaths or longer.
- To come out, lower your knees to the floor. Sit back in Child's Pose (Balasana).

Key Actions

- Be aware of your hands and wrists; there is a tendency to let the palms cup up off the mat. Be sure to press down through all four corners of your palm, especially the base of your index finger and thumb. Keep your forearms long and try to minimize the crease in your wrist by lengthening through your arms and, if necessary, walking your feet farther back. Create a nice long line of energy from the tips of your fingers all the way up each arm.
- To get the most benefit from the pose, it is important to start with a strong foundation. This is true for most poses, but it's particularly important with Downward-Facing Dog Pose. Always check your alignment in the kneeling position until you have a perfect base from which to elongate your spine.

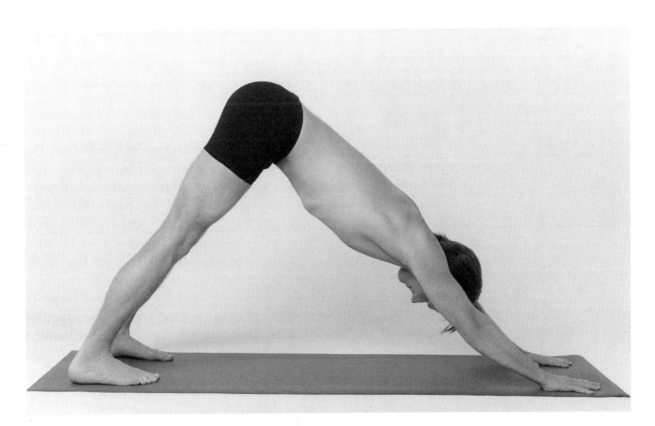

- If your heels reach the floor easily, consider increasing the distance between your hands and feet to increase the stretch. As you lower your heels, imagine a suction cup behind your navel simultaneously lifting your hips higher. This "traction" in your spine helps lengthen the pose.

Modifications

- Beginner: If your hamstrings are tight, bend your knees in the full pose. This will allow the hamstrings to open gently while protecting your lower back.
- Intermediate: Once you are in the full pose, lift your right leg until it forms a straight plane with your torso. Make sure both hips are at the same height. Breathe deeply, and hold for 5 to 10 breaths. Switch legs.
- Advanced: When doing this pose as part of Sun Salutation (Surya Namaskara) and beginning the move into Warrior Pose (Virabhadrasana), draw your extended leg down through your arms and place your foot on the floor in front of your body just between your hands. Do this lightly, without letting your foot drag or stomp.

Benefits

This foundational pose stretches your spine, shoulders, calves, and hamstrings and strengthens your arms, legs, and core. It is also known to relieve headaches.

Contraindications

Do not do this pose if you have wrist issues or high blood pressure.

Inspiration

After years of my own practice, I gained a new appreciation for this pose by watching my own dog! When you see a dog actually move into Downward-Facing Dog Pose, you get to see the pose performed properly. When my dog does this, he moves fluidly, and it's obvious that it feels good. Each time I come into the pose, I think of how he responds, how he really embraces the stretch. He is seldom stagnant but always flowing with the stretch. I allow myself to move around and really feel the fluidity of the pose.

I have observed that, for most of my life, I have told myself what to do. I tell my body how to act, thinking it is good practice for setting up the pose. If you notice that you have this tendency as well, I recommend that you stop giving orders and hollering at your body and instead listen carefully to what it wants from you. During this moment, *experience*. Do not go on autopilot. This is an opportunity to move about and awaken dormant energy that you may not have noticed before.

CHILD'S POSE (BALASANA)

Getting In

- Kneel with your hips stacked over your knees and your shoulders stacked over your hips.
- Bring your big toes together so your lower legs form a V shape.
- Sit back so your buttocks rest on your heels.
- Draw your abdominals in toward your spine.
- Fold forward from your hips without collapsing your spine. Walk your hands out in front of you.
- Your spine and arms should be elongated and parallel but relaxed. Your fingers are splayed, with your palms flat on the floor. Stretch forward from your sit bones, lengthening your spine, neck, and crown.
- With your forehead on your mat, gently press your hips back toward your heels so your pelvis moves toward the floor. Enjoy the stretch in your lower back and thighs.
- Alternatively, you may rest your arms at your sides.
- Close your eyes.
- Breathe deeply.
- Hold for several breaths or longer.
- Return to this restorative pose whenever you feel the need for rejuvenation. It's a good "time out."

Key Actions

- This is a good time to activate your core and prepare for your next pose—or for the day ahead of you. Lengthen your tailbone while opening up your sacrum for a good stretch. Deepen the stretch by drawing your hip bones toward your navel.

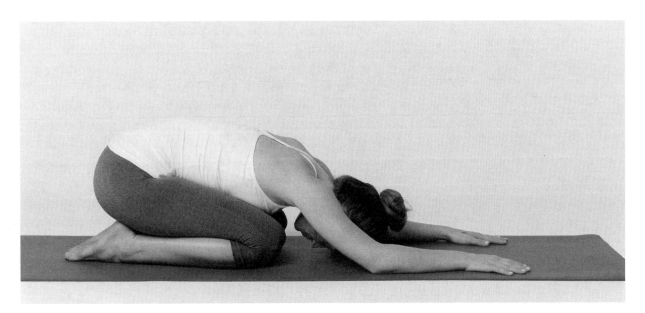

- Breathe consciously into the back of your torso, allowing the breath to lengthen, widen, and soothe your body.
- Do not force your hips back and down, as this can harm your knees. Instead, allow your hips to *relax* back and down to ensure the pose is comfortable and reasonable.

Modifications

- Beginner: If Child's Pose puts unnecessary pressure on the tops of your feet, curl your toes under your heels to lift your feet slightly off the mat. If you are not comfortable in any way, try taking your arms down alongside your body and opening your knees even wider. You can always use some form of support—such as a block, a bolster, or even your hands—under your forehead.
- Intermediate: Alter the pose slightly by keeping your knees together. Rest your torso on your thighs, and ease your buttocks toward your heels. Rest your arms by your sides and your forehead on your mat. Your back will be rounded.

Benefits

This is the main body-calming pose in yoga. It provides a gentle stretch through your hips, thighs, spine, and ankles.

Contraindications

Do not do this pose if you have knee issues or are pregnant.

Inspiration

Child's Pose is a place to restore and return to your breath. Use it as an opportunity to recall any intention you may have set for your practice. It is sometimes tempting to stay a little too long and get too comfortable in this pose, and then you begin to space out and disconnect. But you are here to *reconnect*. So while you may not be working as hard here, be careful to find that place in the middle where you are not only comfortable and restful but also very much awake and focused. If you are in the mood to be in a restorative space, then go for it. If you are incorporating Child's Pose into your flow, sometimes it is good to get back on the road. Otherwise, you are just living at a rest stop. Remember that you will not be in this class or on the mat forever, so try to be efficient and use your time wisely.

CORPSE POSE (SAVASANA)

The Sanskrit name for this pose may also be spelled Shavasana, because in Sanskrit, *shava* means "dead body." To achieve true restorative benefits, you must place both your body and your mind in a state of complete relaxation.

Getting In

- Lie on your back, fully reclined.
- Your hands can be on your belly, palms down, or your arms can be extended alongside your body with your palms up.
- Extend your legs straight out with your feet about shoulder-width apart and turned out slightly.
- Close your eyes.
- Begin to let go of your control over your body and your breath. Your mind should be fully present, observing this deep relaxation taking place.
- Stay here for 5 to 10 minutes or longer.
- To release, bend your knees, roll to the side, and press up to any comfortable seated position. Bring your hands to prayer position.

Key Actions

- Reflect on each part of your body, from your toes all the way up to the crown of your head. Consciously relax each part. Try first tightening each part a little and then releasing and relaxing it. Just let it go.
- Pay attention to your breathing. Rhythmic breathing will help still the mind and put it into a state of deep relaxation, but try not to obsess about the breath. Let go of the powerful Ujjayi Pranayama and allow the breath to relax naturally. In Corpse Pose, you eventually let go of the breath and let your mind be at peace.

Modifications

- Beginner: If your lower back feels discomfort in this pose, roll up a towel or blanket and put it under your knees. You can also bend your knees and place the soles of your feet on the floor.

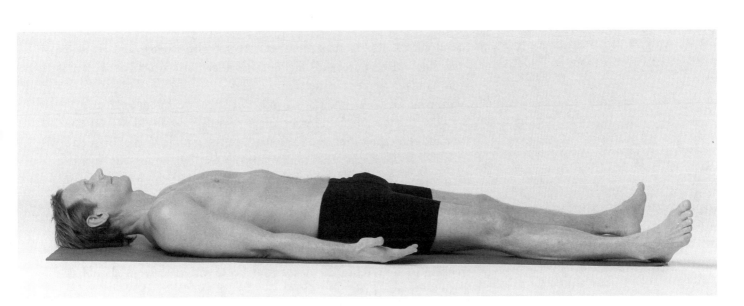

Benefits

This pose calms the mind and balances the body. The deep relaxation helps counter insomnia, nervous disorders, and high blood pressure.

Contraindications

Do not do this pose if you have back issues or are pregnant.

Inspiration

Corpse Pose may seem like the perfect opportunity for figuring out your whole life. It's tempting to use this "downtime" to start planning dinner or work on your five-year life plan. But this is not the time to solve all your problems or to space out and sleep. To experience deep relaxation and get the true benefit of this pose (and of your entire practice), the mind needs to be still yet always aware.

All of the time you spend practicing is worth it when you arrive at a place of rest where you can stop trying to control everything, a place where you can literally just *be*. The body and the breath turn to a natural state of relaxation. The mind is your observer. If you are spacing out and not present, you do not know if your breath is cut off from your experience. Allow everything to be as it is. Be present and let go of your breath and body. Giving yourself this precious time for rejuvenation is one of the kindest things you can do for yourself, your family, and your community.

Mountain Pose (Tadasana)

Mountain Pose is the foundation for all standing poses. Master it first, and you will create a beautiful foundation for every other standing asana.

Getting In

- Stand with your big toes together, heels slightly apart, and arms at your sides with your palms facing in. You can also do this pose with your hands in prayer position.
- Align your hips over your knees and your knees over your ankles.
- Set your foundation. Bend your knees slightly, pressing down on one foot and then the other. Find the space in the middle of each foot and evenly distribute your weight between your feet. Maintain your balance by pressing your feet into the floor. Contract your thigh muscles for support and lift the arches of your feet.
- Find your center. Focus on the area around your navel. Inhale as you lengthen your lower back, sending your tailbone down as you lift the front of your pelvis. Draw in your abdominal muscles. Align your spine, stacking each vertebra. Elongate your neck, and lower your shoulders away from your ears.

- Feel the energy flowing from your toes up through your legs to the crown of your head and back down through your fingertips and toes.
- Draw your shoulder blades down and toward each other, and open your chest.
- Direct your gaze straight ahead.
- Breathe deeply. Hold for 5 to 10 breaths or longer.

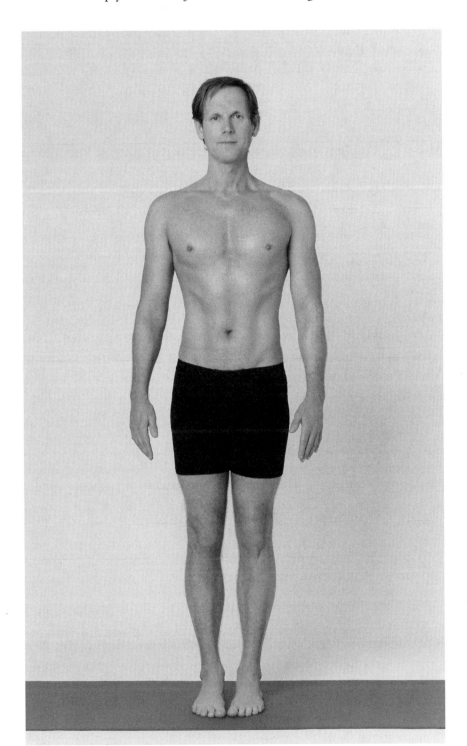

Key Actions

- Starting from the ground up, make sure your big toes are touching, your anklebones are slightly apart, and your thighs are rotated slightly inward. Some schools dictate that your feet should be apart, but to me, it doesn't matter. I love honoring tradition and breaking it too.

Modifications

- Beginner: If you are pregnant or feel more comfortable with the feet wider apart, move the feet hip-width to find a stable and grounded sense of balance.

Benefits

Mountain Pose lets you return to your inherent state of equanimity: steady, strong, and soft. You are able to experience a moment without struggle. There is action, but there is no stress or worry.

Contraindications

Do not do this pose if you have low blood pressure or a headache.

Inspiration

I like Mountain Pose, which is also called Samasthiti. It represents an energetic space as well as a moment when you have been called home, invited to remember what this practice is really about. When I come to Mountain Pose, I do not get sloppy or casual. It is a state of accepting that I am right where I need to be. There must be courage in the heart to see this. I am enveloped by present-time awareness. I am honoring my duty.

Mountain Pose sets the foundation for all standing poses. It is a great place to begin your practice. Like Staff Pose (Dandasana; page 196), which sets a foundation for seated poses, Mountain Pose helps to establish intention and set your alignment. A lot of folks think, "I'm just standing up. It's no big deal." But, it *is* a big deal. It is a foundation of your yoga practice.

Standing Forward Bend (Uttanasana)

Getting In

- Start in Mountain Pose (Tadasana), with your feet together.
- Bend your knees slightly; fold your torso over your legs; and let your head and arms dangle, relaxed, toward the floor in front of your toes.
- Rest your palms at the sides of your feet, bending your knees as much as necessary to get there. Relax your spine and shoulders.
- Exhale. Feel your upper body getting heavier and your head falling closer to the floor.

- Place your hands on your ankles or shins. On an inhalation, straighten your knees and arms to lift your torso halfway, reaching your spine forward. Stretch your quadricep muscles, and lengthen your spine. This is Standing Half Forward Bend (Ardha Uttanasana). Go back down on the exhalation.
- On an exhalation, fold your torso back down and draw your torso and head toward your straight legs, putting your hands on the floor.
- Hold for 5 to 10 breaths or longer.
- To release, bend your knees and roll back up, vertebra by vertebra, into Mountain Pose.

Key Actions

- Your feet can be as wide apart as your head, or you can bring them together. If you do open your feet, make sure your hips are stacked over your heels.
- Try to place your palms flat on the mat. I recommend bending your knees enough to make this happen and keeping them bent. If you can

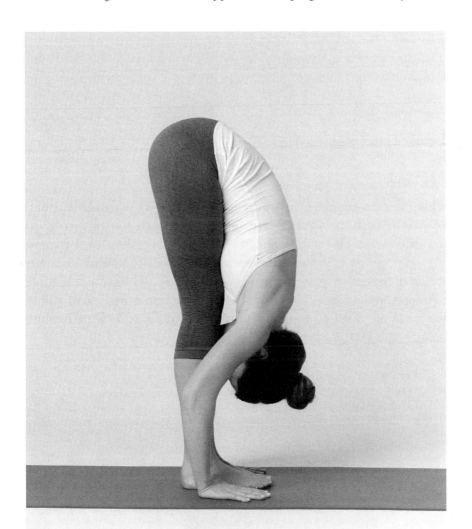

straighten your legs by hinging at your hips while keeping your palms on the floor, cool; but try not to push your thighs backward. Instead, lift your hips toward the sky and then straighten your legs.

- Bring your weight forward onto the balls of your feet.
- If the base of your palms starts to lift off the mat, you have straightened your legs too much. Work on drawing your navel in and pressing the heels of your palms down. This is how to gauge the degree to which you can safely straighten your legs.
- A wonderful way to approach this fold is to hinge from your hips, not your lower back. This way, you elongate your spine instead of rounding your back. Be sure your hands remain soft, with your fingers relaxed and not gripping the floor. The action, once again, is in your legs.

Modifications

- Beginner: If the floor is very far away, you can use two blocks to bring it up to meet you. Place the blocks in front of your feet to support your hands.

Benefits

This pose stretches your spine, hamstrings, calves, hips, and torso. It also strengthens your spine and thighs.

Contraindications

Do not do this pose if you have back or neck issues.

Inspiration

This pose is an exercise in offering and surrendering. We are surrendering to what we perceive is our current duty in our lives. It is a willing surrender. No one is telling us or forcing us to do anything. We are not victims. We are empowered to give in and trust. Let the pose be a friend, a teacher we listen to, not an enemy that is hollering at us. Let this be a moment of inquiry and intrigue, a moment to claim the power that resides within the act of surrendering without ever being submissive. We are active and participating. We choose to be here.

CHAPTER 9

Standing Poses

Standing poses are a great place to discover strength and support from the ground up. Building more power in these poses helps us move through everyday life with more ease, assurance, and stability. Building this strength from the feet up through the legs also brings strength to the core and upper body.

When we develop focus during these exercises, we can take that ability to concentrate with us into our daily interactions. These poses give us self-confidence and an ability to navigate sudden changes in life.

CROUCHING WARRIOR POSE—LOW POSITION

Getting In

- Start in a lunge position with your right foot forward and your left foot behind. Bend your right knee at a 90-degree angle. Tuck your left toes under and lift your left knee off the floor. Place your fingertips or palms on your mat on either side of your right foot.
- Move the fingers of your right hand to your right hip crease and the fingers of your left hand to the top of your right foot. Keep your spine long and draw your navel toward your spine. Avoid twisting to either side.
- Bring your chest slightly forward and up as you stand firmly on your right foot. Keep your right knee bent as you lift your left leg, bringing it parallel to the floor behind you. Your chest should also be parallel to the floor.
- Keep your chest lifting away from your right thigh, and make sure your neck is long (a true extension of your spine).
- Rotate your left thigh inward and aim your toes toward the floor as you level your hips.

- Direct your gaze straight down at the floor.
- Breathe deeply.
- Hold for several breaths or longer.
- To release, carefully lower back to a lunge position and return your hands to the mat on either side of your right foot. Switch legs and repeat, or continue on to Crouching Warrior Pose—Up Position.

Key Actions

- Maintain a long line of energy from the toes of your lifted leg through that hip, your spine, and the crown of your head. There is no twisting action in this pose.
- Keep your front knee bent and activate Uddiyana Bandha (Abdominal Lock) to keep your chest lifted off the thigh of your standing leg.
- Use the fingers in your hip crease to encourage the hip to stay lifted and drawn back slightly.

Modifications

- Beginner: If you have knee issues, keep your front knee straight and work on building strength around the knee. If it is difficult to maintain your balance, place the fingers of your left hand on the floor just inside your right foot for support.

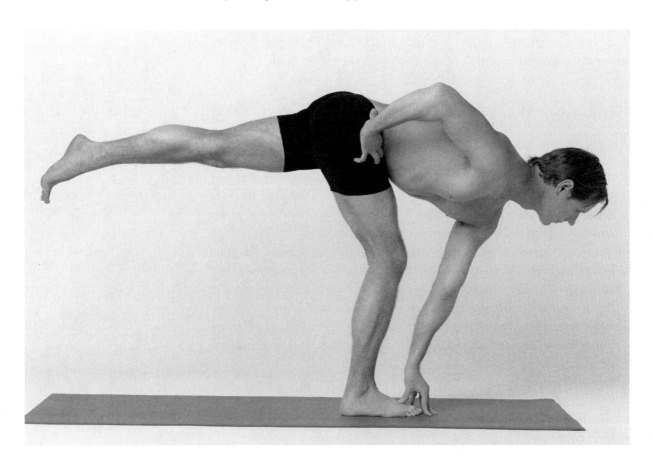

- Intermediate: To build even more strength in your quadriceps, hips, and gluteal muscles, try bending (on an inhalation) and straightening (on an exhalation) your front knee. Keep your hips level, your back leg parallel to the floor, and your spine long as you lift and lower in this challenging but rewarding position.

Benefits

A long line of energy will support you as you strengthen and tone your abdominals, hips, glutes, and legs.

Contraindications

Do not do this pose if you have knee issues.

Inspiration

Like Virabhadrasana III (Warrior III Pose), this asana relies on the strength of the standing leg and the squaring of the hips to maintain balance. However, with the standing knee bent, the front foot and ankle have to work hard. When you stay in the pose, your quads and glutes suddenly kick in to take over some of the effort. Hold your stance! The tendency here is to allow the mind to take over and want to straighten the standing leg. Do not give in. Keep your knee bent; stay committed to building your strength; and focus on your deep, rhythmic breath.

CROUCHING WARRIOR POSE—UP POSITION

Getting In

- Start in Crouching Warrior Pose—Low Position, with your right knee bent and your left leg long behind you. The fingers of your right hand are in your right hip crease and the fingers of your left are on top of your right foot.
- Bring your left hand to your left hip.
- Bend your left knee in toward your chest and the heel toward your left buttock.
- Press firmly into your right foot. Do not let your left foot touch the ground as you rise to standing with your left knee lifted toward your chest.
- Straighten your right leg slightly as you lift your left knee even higher. Lift the center of your chest toward the sky as you drop your tailbone toward the floor. You are now in a standing position with your knee in toward your chest.
- Keep a slight bend in your standing knee.
- Direct your gaze straight out in front of you.
- Breathe deeply.

- Hold for several breaths or longer.
- Return to Crouching Warrior Pose—Low Position by bending your right knee as you lower your chest halfway down. Maintain the length in your spine.
- Send your left leg back out behind you, parallel to the floor. Lower the fingers of your left hand to your right foot.
- Repeat this cycle of rising to Up Position and descending to Low Position several times.

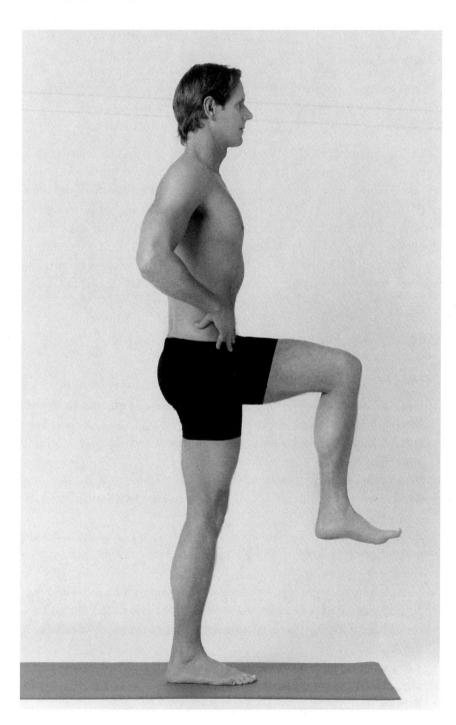

- To release from Low Position, carefully lower your left toes back to a lunge position and return your hands to the mat on either side of your right foot. Change sides.

Key Actions

- As you rise to standing, focus on keeping your lifted knee as close to your chest as possible. Activate Uddiyana Bandha (Abdominal Lock) to help keep your foot off the ground.
- Once you are standing, strengthen your standing leg by drawing the kneecap up without locking your knee.
- While moving between Up and Low positions, keep your standing leg bent to build even more strength in the entire leg, hip, and glute.

Benefits

This pose strengthens and tones your abdominals, hips, glutes, and legs.

Contraindications

Do not do this pose if you have knee issues. Instead, remain in Low Position and keep your standing leg straight. Stay here and build strength around the knee.

Inspiration

The hardest thing about this pose is often the sense of fatigue students feel in the standing foot and leg. Even the movement up and down is a lot of work. After students practice these variations of Warrior Pose (Virabhadrasana), it makes the other Warrior poses seem easy by contrast. Core, hip, and total leg strength are all required to maintain and move between these positions, but most important, it takes absolute concentration to do this work. This is one of the most challenging sequences, but often the times of great challenge in our lives bring the greatest amount of growth and reward.

LUNGE POSE VARIATION

This is a great preparation for Warrior I Pose (Virabhadrasana I), but it's also a fine pose on its own.

Getting In

- Start in Downward-Facing Dog Pose (Adho Mukha Svanasana).
- Step your right foot forward, placing it flat on the mat between your hands. Your right knee should be at a 90-degree angle and aligned over your ankle.
- Straighten your left leg completely and engage your left thigh.

- Your left heel should be off the ground. Lengthen the pose by pressing back through your left heel.
- Lift your torso and arms to vertical. Extend your arms up beside your ears with the palms facing each other.
- Realign your posture. Send your tailbone down and engage your abdominal muscles. Stretch all the way through the crown of your head, feeling your spine extend away from your pelvis.
- Direct your gaze forward.

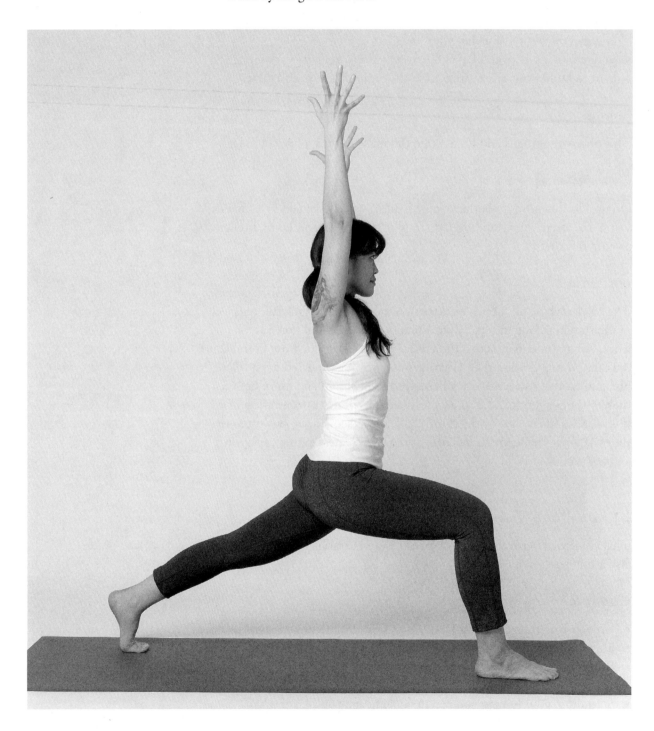

- Breathe deeply. Hold for 5 to 10 breaths or longer.
- Release to Downward-Facing Dog Pose.
- Switch legs and repeat.

Key Actions

- Check your alignment. The outside edge of your front foot should be parallel to the edge of the mat. Your bent knee is over your ankle.
- Seek out a sense of lightness in your hips. Let them move down toward the floor, while simultaneously imagining the base of your pelvis lifting.
- Your core should be engaged, and there is no compression in your spine.
- Your back heel is lifted and squared off; your back toes are curled under. Try not to let your back foot collapse inward. Make sure the baby toe is participating, whether or not it touches the earth. (It will be excited that you thought about it.)

Modifications

- Beginner: Most of us do not want to stay in this pose for long, so do some dips instead. Let your lower knee drop to hover about two inches from the floor, hold for several breaths, straighten both legs, and then bend just the front knee again. Repeat a few times. Dips are invigorating. Adding a few can awaken your core energy and keep you from getting sloppy. You can also modify your arms by placing your hands on your hips or bringing your hands into prayer position (Anjali Mudra).
- Intermediate: Interlace your fingers behind your back.

Benefits

In one fell swoop, you can enjoy a good stretch in your knees, hamstrings, thighs, and spine while strengthening your arms and shoulders.

Contraindications

Do not do this pose if you have heart issues. If you have high blood pressure, modify the pose by bringing your back knee to the mat and your hands to your hips or to prayer position at your heart.

Inspiration

Do not engage in a tug-of-war with your body. It is easy to overstretch in this pose. There is the temptation to let the full force of your body lunge forward into the pose and overstretch the groin and thigh muscles, a delicate area to overwork. To avoid injury, be sure to control your lunge and listen to your body as your legs, groins, and hips move in opposite directions.

HAND UNDER FOOT POSE (PADAHASTHASANA)

Getting In

- Start in Mountain Pose (Tadasana), with your hips squared.
- Position your feet hip- or head-width apart. Be sure the outside edges of your feet are parallel to the sides of your mat.
- Place your hands on your hips.
- Engage your core, bend forward from your hips, and bring your torso parallel to the floor. Keep your spine straight; bend your knees if necessary. Pause long enough to feel the full extension of the spine.
- Continue into a full forward fold, placing your hands beside your feet. Place your palms or your fingertips on the ground.
- From the front of your feet, slide the palms of your hands face up under the balls of your feet. Walk your toes close to your wrist creases so your feet are lightly resting on your hands.
- Bend your elbows out to the sides and use the strength of your biceps to draw yourself deeper into the fold. Let your head hang heavy, keeping your neck relaxed.

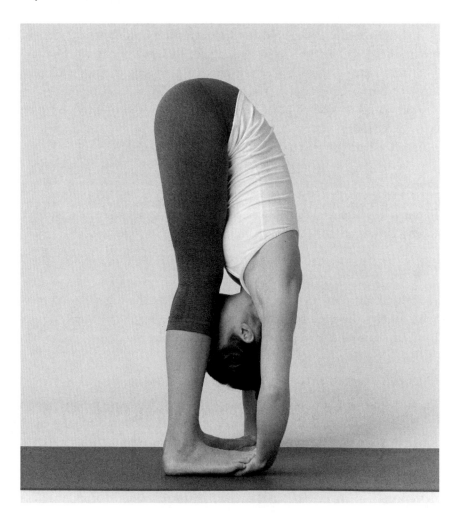

- Inhale as you draw your head and neck up to knee height. Direct your gaze forward. Elongate your neck. Press your hands toward the floor, and lengthen your spine.
- Exhale as you fold your head, neck, and torso back down.
- Guide your shoulders toward your hips and away from your ears.
- Hold for 5 to 10 breaths or longer.
- To release, bring your hands to your hips, engage your core, and rise back up to Mountain Pose.

Key Actions

- Bring your weight forward until there is a slight pressure on your hands and your forearms engage.
- Give yourself permission to move into this pose honestly and safely by bending your knees. As your legs straighten, begin to engage your thighs.

Modification

- Beginner: If this pose feels too deep, bring your hands to your shins or bend your knees more. Find a level of comfort that is suitable for you. Do not proceed to the full pose until you are ready.

Benefits

This pose stretches your hamstrings, calves, and spine and strengthens your legs.

Contraindications

Do not do this pose if you have wrist or lower back issues.

Inspiration

Giving yourself permission to bend your knees can make a big difference in your practice, particularly in your forward bends. Build the pose over time by backing off and trying to honor this one simple detail of alignment. The stretch may go farther and improve faster if you back off in the beginning. It is also a lot safer. By forcing your body into deep stretches before it is ready, your risk of injury becomes significantly greater.

BIG TOE POSE (PADANGUSTHASANA)

Getting In

- Start in Mountain Pose (Tadasana), with your hips squared.
- Position your feet hip- or head-width apart. Be sure the outside edges of your feet are parallel to the sides of your mat.

- Place your hands on your hips.
- Engage your core, bend forward from your hips, and bring your torso parallel to the floor. Keep your spine straight by bending the knees if necessary. Pause long enough to feel the full extension of the spine.
- Continue into a full forward bend, placing your hands beside your feet. Place your palms or fingertips on the floor.
- Wrap your index and middle fingers around your big toes from the inside.
- Bend your elbows and use the strength of your biceps to draw yourself deeper into the fold. Let your head hang heavy, keeping your neck relaxed.
- Inhale as you draw your head and neck up to knee height. Direct your gaze forward. Elongate your neck. Press your hands toward the floor, and lengthen your spine.
- Exhale as you fold your head, neck, and torso back down.
- Guide your shoulders toward your hips and away from your ears.
- Hold for 5 to 10 breaths or longer.

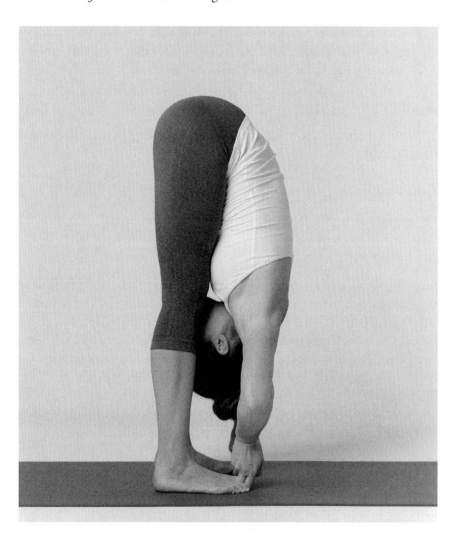

- To release, bring your hands to your hips, engage your core, and come back up to Mountain Pose.

Key Actions

- Hold your big toes. We are often told to keep our feet "hip-width apart," but many students think their hips are wider than they actually are. In reality, your feet should only be about 8 to 10 inches apart. Your ears should fit exactly between your legs. This provides an honest and accessible distance between your feet. Stack your hips over your heels.
- I am a big knee bender. I love to do it in every forward fold, bringing my hips slightly forward. With my knees bent, I notice that I can hinge farther from my hips, bringing more of my weight into the balls of my feet, which effectively invites more length in my lower back. There is a tendency here to try to force your legs to straighten by pushing your knees back and bringing your weight into your heels, which creates an extra stretch behind your knee instead of in the healthy, core part of the hamstring.
- Do not grip with your toes. Feel the arches of your feet awaken.

Modification

- Beginner: If it is too challenging to take hold of your big toes, you can simply place your hands on your shins or even take your fingers around your elbows. Be sure to hinge forward from your hips. Your back should be straight.

Benefits

When done with grace, this pose gently stretches your hamstrings, calves, and the backs of your knees. It simultaneously strengthens your thighs, legs, and ankles.

Contraindications

Do not do this pose if you have neck or lower back issues.

Inspiration

I often meet students who think they have to straighten their legs no matter how rounded their spine is. Revert to a beginner's mind; instead of thinking of straightening your legs, think of pressing your heels down and lifting your hips straight up. Bending your knees can make a big difference in your practice. Students who take this advice develop splendid alignment.

Parivritta Parsvakonasana (Revolved Side-Angle Pose)

Getting In

- Start in Downward-Facing Dog Pose (Adho Mukha Svanasana).
- Step your right foot forward between your hands.
- Drop your hips slightly lower than your right knee. Activate your quadriceps and hamstrings. Direct your gaze forward and down.
- Inhale as you lift your arms. Align your arms with your ears, with the palms facing each other.
- Spin your left heel around to a 45-degree angle and press into the heel. Draw in your navel and lengthen your tailbone.
- Bring your palms together at your heart. Inhale and lift your heart.
- As you exhale, rotate your torso to the right so you are twisting toward your front leg.
- Hook the tricep of your left (bottom) arm outside your right (front) thigh.
- Your right elbow should point toward the sky.
- Press your palms together to deepen the twist.
- Your hips should be square with the floor. Turn from the base of your spine. Hug your navel against your right thigh.
- Create a long, straight line from the outer edge of your back heel through the crown of your head. As you deepen the stretch, this line of energy becomes even more revitalizing.
- Breathe deeply. Hold for 5 to 10 breaths or longer.
- Release by reversing out of the pose.
- Repeat on the other side.

Key Actions

- If moving into the twist causes the rest of your alignment to collapse, back off a bit and reestablish a solid foundation.
- There is a strong desire to bind, but if you lose the line of energy from your sacrum to the crown of your head, then you are closing off the connection with the opening of *sushumna nadi*. Liberate your central axis by maintaining long and open lines of energy.

Modifications

- Beginner: If spinning your back heel down constricts your breath or causes any discomfort in the knee, lift your heel back up and remain on the ball of your back foot. Maintain a sense of Uddiyana Bandha (Abdominal Lock) in the twist, trying to lift your navel up and past your thigh. Lighten up on the twist.
- Intermediate: Once you are in the twist with hands in prayer position, keep the rotation of your torso but open your arms. Place your

left palm on the floor at the outer edge of your right foot. Reach your right arm straight up toward the sky. Rotate your torso and top arm to the right until your chest is fully open to the right side. Reach through both arms.

Benefits

Let the lines of energy enhance the stretches through your abdominal and groin muscles, spine, and shoulders. This pose strengthens your ankles, knees, and legs.

Contraindications

Do not do this pose if you have a headache, high or low blood pressure, or insomnia.

Inspiration

I see folks trying so hard to become picture perfect and missing the experience of letting this pose find them. I love the beginner's state of curiosity, borne out of both asking and listening to the body and the mind. Oftentimes, because of a sense of routine, this special experience might

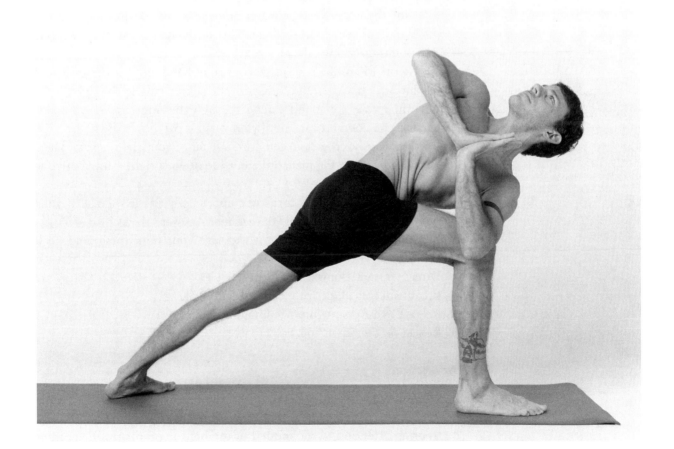

be overlooked by more seasoned practitioners. So, pause, back off, and simply breathe into the moment at hand. That is a more mature state. Feel a sense of both hips lifting a little instead of letting one collapse. Bring buoyancy into the pose.

The key is maintaining the long line of energy from your back heel to the crown of your head. This can determine if you need to go deeper or back off. Use your core. It is the obliques (outer abdominal muscles) that twist the torso. Let your obliques help you; do not just use your shoulders. Your head only turns as a healthy consequence of the twist. Don't yank it to the side. Your neck is the last thing to turn. You can even turn your gaze down to deflect any temptation to overtwist your neck.

REVOLVED TRIANGLE POSE (PARIVRITTA TRIKONASANA)

Getting In

- Start in Mountain Pose (Tadasana).
- Inhale and step your left foot behind you about three or four feet. Position your feet so they would be about hip-width apart if they were side-by-side, rather than one in front of the other—but remember, not too wide. Turn your left foot out to a 45-degree angle, with your left heel touching the floor. Keep your right foot at the top of the mat, with the outer edge of your foot parallel to the outer edge of the mat and your toes pointing straight ahead.
- Facing the top of the mat, place your right hand on your right hip and reach your left arm straight up, with the palm facing to the right.
- Lengthen your spine and extend through the fingertips of your left hand as you bend forward until your torso is parallel to the floor.
- Simultaneously, cross your left arm in front of your right leg and place your left hand on the mat to the outside of your right foot, with your fingertips pointing forward.
- Keeping your hips level, turn your upper body to the right. Lift your right shoulder, then extend your right arm toward the sky.
- Enjoy the horizontal stretch. Make sure your hips, torso, and neck are aligned.
- Direct your gaze upward.
- Breathe deeply. Hold for 5 to 10 breaths or longer.
- Release by reversing into Mountain Pose.
- Repeat on the other side.

Key Actions

- Alignment is crucial in Revolved Triangle Pose. Check to see if your weight is drifting to the lateral (outside) part of your front foot. Try to bring attention to the mound of the big toe on that foot, creating a deeper arch and trying to balance between the mound of the big toe and the inner heel.

- Also pay attention to your back foot, pressing it down and to the midline. Some yoga enthusiasts are so gung ho about creating a deeper twist that they end up weakening and overstretching the outer back ankle. Focus on creating safer footing for the long haul by first establishing a firm foundation.

- Be strong in both legs, pressing both heels down into the floor and allowing your right hip to move back as your left hip moves slightly forward. Your hips are always squared forward.

- Squeeze your inner thighs together and engage your core to create a lifting and lengthening sensation from your hips and lower back.

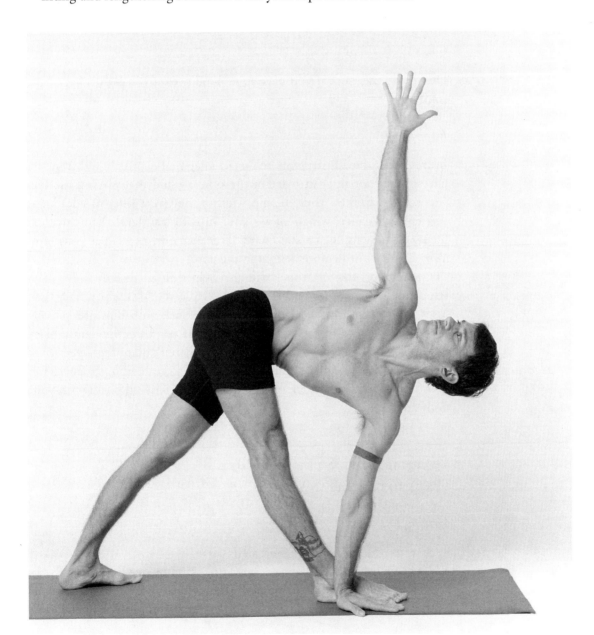

Modification

- Beginner: If you are having problems touching the floor without collapsing your spine, place a block on the inside (to start) or the outside (later on) of your front foot. Lower your hand to the block. Or place your hand on the floor just inside or on top of your front foot. Place your upper hand on your sacrum. This will allow you to feel if your hips are level.

Benefits

Maintaining the alignment in this pose ensures a safe stretch through your groins, hamstrings, hips, and spine. It also strengthens your legs and twists through your core.

Contraindications

Do not do this pose if you have low blood pressure, a headache, or insomnia.

Inspiration

In this pose, some instructors tell us to imagine being on a tightrope by having one foot right in front of the other. I find that placing the feet wider apart (so they would be hip-width if they were side-by-side) helps you create balance, which allows your hips to stay level. You can then focus on enjoying the twist. Open your stance only as wide as your hips. You will find a little more delight in the pose.

Getting "off the tightrope" will also help with balance if you've been struggling. A common tendency is to collapse the back hip, which then loses the strength of the hamstring. Make sure both hips are actively pressing back toward the wall behind you. If you can confidently place your opposite hand down, good work. If you aren't quite there yet, that's fine too. Don't spend your short time in this pose battling balance. Let go of the struggle and back off to find a more balanced position in your body and mind.

Intense Side Stretch Pose (Parsvottanasana)

Getting In

- Start in Mountain Pose (Tadasana).
- Move your hands into reverse prayer position by bending your elbows behind your back and drawing your hands toward the center. Tilt your torso forward for a moment to increase the flexibility in your arms.

Turn your palms to face each other, and bring the fingers and then the palms together in prayer position. With your fingers pointing toward the sky, gently slide your hands up between your shoulder blades.

- Inhale and step your left foot, staggered, behind you about three or four feet. Like the last pose, keep your feet about hip-width apart, not "on a tightrope."
- Turn your left foot out to a 45-degree angle, with your left heel pressing down into the floor.
- Square your hips toward the front of the mat.
- Wiggle your spine and shoulders to release any tension. As you inhale, lengthen and lift your spine. Keep your shoulders relaxed.
- Fold forward over your legs until your torso is just parallel to the floor. Press your heels down into the floor and keep moving your hips back, maintaining a long spine. Press your hands closer together behind you, opening your chest.
- Continue to bend forward until your chest is resting on your thigh.
- Direct your gaze toward the toes of your right foot. If that is uncomfortable for your neck, keep your neck long and gaze down toward your right leg.
- Breathe deeply. Hold for 5 to 10 breaths or longer.
- To release, reverse back to Mountain Pose. Reverse legs and repeat on the other side.

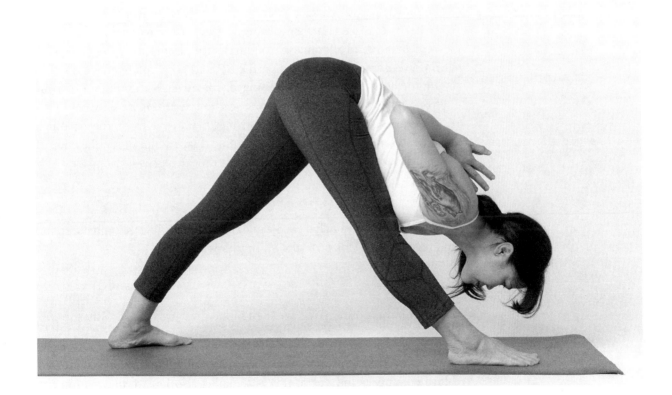

Key Actions

- Use your core as you come back up, lifting your chest and adding a slight backbend. Activating your core maintains life in the pose. Press your back heel away from your torso. Make sure both hips are drawn back as well.
- Lower halfway down until your chest is parallel to the floor. It can be a lot more challenging and exhilarating to hold here for a few breaths, keeping everything activated while drawing length into your spine. After a few breaths, determine whether or not you would benefit from folding deeper into the pose, always maintaining a strong core in order to protect your lower back.
- When you lean too much to one side, the pose becomes vulnerable. Develop strength in this pose by creating a long, beautiful line, not only through your spine, but also through both sides of your body.
- Let the hip of your back leg drop down to experience a really good hamstring stretch while protecting the side of your lower back through solid alignment. If you are not allowing for a good hamstring stretch, you are in the wrong pose. There is no denying that this is a leg-strengthening exercise. While your spine, hips, core, shoulders, and wrists are all working in this pose, your leg muscles have to be the strongest and the most comprehensively engaged.

Modifications

- Beginner: If you can keep your hands in reverse prayer position, great. Otherwise, place your hands wherever necessary to retain support for your breath and alignment. You might try placing them on your hips. Both feet are firmly planted on the floor to keep you from leaning too far to the side. Consider pressing down through the mound of your front big toe and your front inner heel to create this stability.
- Beginner: If you have tight hamstrings, bend your front knee as much as necessary to gain length in your spine. Place a block on either side of your front foot and let your hands rest on the blocks for support.

Benefits

Activating your core helps you get a deep stretch in your shoulders, spine, and hamstrings. This pose also strengthens your legs.

Contraindications

Do not do this pose if you have high blood pressure or back issues.

Inspiration

I love coming in and out of this pose, and I also love to play within the pose. Sometimes coming out of it a little and not going so deep (leaving your chest halfway down versus trying to get your head all the way down) is very interesting. I personally prefer keeping the head no lower than the chest, because when pressing your forehead beyond where your chest can go, you overstretch the back of your neck and create a crease in your neck (neither of which is healthy). Keep a long line from your lower back through to the crown of your head.

WIDE-LEGGED FORWARD BEND (PRASARITA PADOTTANASANA)

Getting In

- Start in Mountain Pose (Tadasana).
- Step your feet about three to four feet apart, and turn your toes in slightly so your heels are a bit wider apart than your toes.
- Place your hands on your hips.
- Find your center. Press your feet down into the floor to activate your legs and core. Feel the energy rise up through your legs and navel. Lengthen your tailbone and send the energy back down your legs.
- Fold your torso forward and place your hands flat on the floor shoulder-distance apart between your feet. The crown of your head should be facing the floor, and it may or may not touch the mat.
- Inhale and straighten your arms, raise your chest and head, look forward; lengthen your torso.
- Exhale and allow your head to drop as you fold forward deeply. Walk your hands back until your fingertips are in line with your big toes.
- Your head, neck, and spine should be in one vertical line. As your spine lengthens, your head inches closer to the floor. Bend your elbows as your head drops. If the crown of your head easily touches the ground, bring your feet closer together to create more distance for your spine to lengthen.
- Direct your gaze straight back between your legs.
- Breathe deeply. Hold for 5 to 10 breaths or longer.
- To release, place your hands on your hips and raise your torso back to an upright position.

Key Actions

- Go for the stretch. With your feet slightly pigeon-toed, you may feel the stretch in various parts of your legs. Breathe into the deepest part of the stretch.
- I love to play with this pose. I encourage students to bend one knee slightly, then the other, and then both at the same time. From this bent-knee position, try not to drift too far back into your heels as you begin to straighten your legs. Notice how this affects your forward fold.

- Place your weight forward into the balls of your feet. Once (and if) you establish the flexibility, straight legs become the strength and foundation of this pose; they are the ultimate focus here. Help set up a solid foundation so you can eventually find the tilt of your pelvis.
- With your hands down, palms on the floor, and fingers and thumbs splayed, allow the crown of your head to move toward the floor. Keep your spine and neck as long as possible. If you find yourself rounding your back in an effort to place your head on the ground, you have lost the essence of the pose.

Modifications

- Beginner: If your head does not easily reach the floor, consider resting it lightly on a block so you can relax into the stretch in your legs. If you want to explore, open your feet wider or bring them closer together. Notice how it affects the stretch. Find the place where you encounter the most challenge while still feeling safe.
- Intermediate: In forward folds, enjoy the extra stretching behind your knees. If you are already supple and do not need any additional flexibility there, bend your knees and contract your hamstrings to build strength behind your thighs. This requires self-awareness.
- Advanced: One arm variation is to clasp your hands behind your back and lift your arms over your head. As you bring your arms over, they will form a triangle behind your head. Try pressing your palms together, lengthen through your arms, and enjoy the shoulder stretch.

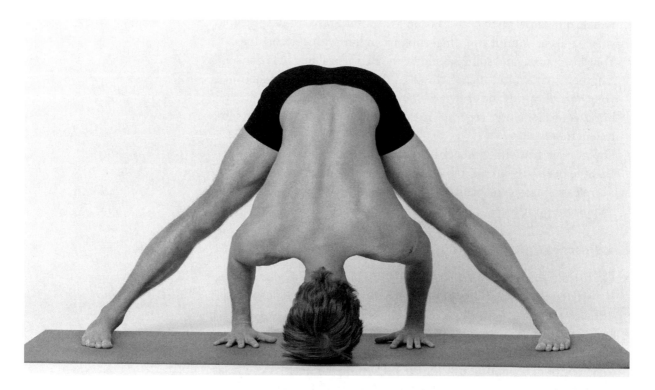

Benefits

You can expand the stretch through your hamstrings, groins, thighs, shoulders, and spine.

Contraindications

Do not do this pose if you have lower back issues.

Inspiration

If you are at the point where you space out because you are so flexible, you are not practicing yoga anymore. Yoga is about feeling something and acknowledging it in the moment, allowing it to be as it is. It is paying attention. If you are thinking, *Look at me. I'm so stretchy, I don't have to work in this pose*, then you have abandoned the true significance of the practice.

CHAIR POSE (UTKATASANA)

Getting In

- Stand in Mountain Pose (Tadasana).
- Inhale as you raise your arms above your head, palms facing in. If it is comfortable for your shoulders, draw the palms of your hands together. Tilt your head up slightly to gaze at your hands.
- Breathe deeply.
- Exhale and bend your knees, leaning your torso forward at a 45-degree angle. Lower your sit bones as if you are going to sit down in a chair. Keep shifting your weight back into your heels.
- Draw on your core to maintain a strong foundation, keeping your core, neck, and head on one plane. There is a natural curve in the low back, but try not to overemphasize this. Instead, think of sending your tailbone down in order to extend the spine. Elongate your neck.
- Press your feet evenly into the floor. Keep your weight evenly distributed through your feet, both side-to-side and back to front.
- Direct your gaze forward or up toward your hands.
- Breathe deeply. Hold for 5 to 10 breaths or longer.
- Release by returning to Mountain Pose.

Key Actions

- Activate your legs and core equally, asking your body to dip down and lift up at the same time. Sink your hips back and down, but keep your heart lifted. This pose is not only about your legs. It is about the wonderful partnership between your core and your legs.

- You do not have to dip terribly low to get a stretch in your glutes and quads. The intensity of this deceptively challenging pose is why I both love it and hate it.

Modifications

- Beginner: Rest your hands on your upper thighs to relieve tension in your upper legs and groins.
- Intermediate: Lift your heels slightly and feel how it engages even more leg power. Hold 5 to 10 breaths.

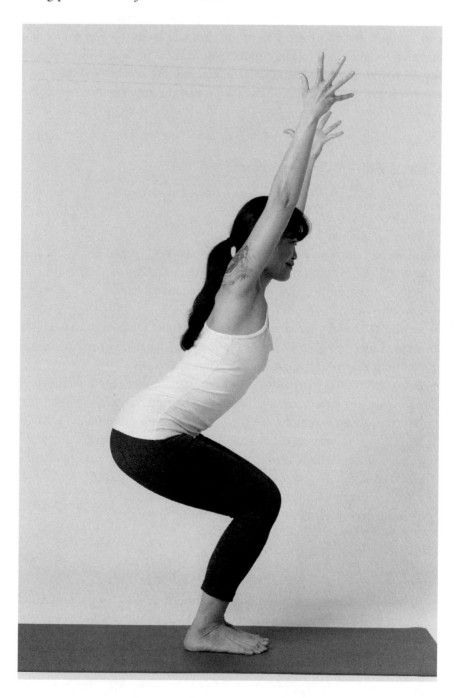

Benefits

Sit back and enjoy the stretch in your glutes, quads, shoulders, and chest. This pose strengthens your ankles, calves, spine, and lower back.

Contraindications

Do not do this pose if you have a headache, insomnia, or low blood pressure.

Inspiration

This pose is a perfect example of how practicing yoga on your mat can prepare you for times in your life when you may need to draw on the strength you have created here. Chair Pose builds more strength in your lower extremities and in your core. Building and maintaining strength in these areas now will help you as you get older and begin to experience the muscle atrophy and reduced flexibility that comes with age. When you get older, you will still be able to pick up anything you might drop.

I have renamed this asana Pleasure Pose. Instead of calling it "Awkward Squat," I encourage people to find something that gives them pleasure in this pose. I see students' attitudes change immediately. They manage to find a moment of fun, and their perspective shifts.

EXTENDED SIDE-ANGLE POSE (UTTHITA PARSVAKONASANA)

Getting In

- Start in Warrior II Pose (Virabhadrasana II; page 114) with your right leg forward.
- Hinge laterally to the right from your hips, and place your right forearm on your right thigh, palm up.
- Extend your left arm over your ear so that the fingertips point toward the front of the mat and the palm faces down. Stretch through your left side, from the outer edge of your left foot through the fingertips of your left hand.
- Lower your right hand to the floor on the inside of your right foot, with your fingertips or palm on the mat. Press your right elbow against the inside of your right knee for support. Keep your knee stacked directly over your ankle and your weight distributed evenly on your right foot, making sure to press down on the outside of that foot.
- Turn your head toward your left arm.
- Slowly rotate your chest and navel toward the sky with each breath.
- You can direct your gaze up, straight ahead, or down at the floor.
- Breathe deeply. Hold for 5 to 10 breaths or longer.
- Release by lifting back up into Warrior II Pose.
- Reverse legs and repeat on the other side.

Key Actions

- Make certain your stance is long enough to ensure that your front knee does not extend beyond the ankle. The knee should form a clean 90-degree angle.
- The foundation is in your bent leg, with that knee stacked over your heel. Never let your knee splay to either side; keep it centered. At the same time, your back leg stays active.
- Explore bringing your lower hand to the outside of your front foot instead of the inside. By playing with these two different pose variations, you can find the one that allows you to create the longer line of energy. Allow your bottom shoulder to press gently into your leg while your leg presses gently back into your shoulder. Go back and forth. It is subtle, but it is dynamic. Notice the difference in the action of your legs as your hand position changes. If at any point it becomes too intense and you notice your breath becoming restricted, modify by bringing your forearm back up to your thigh; this should free up your breath.

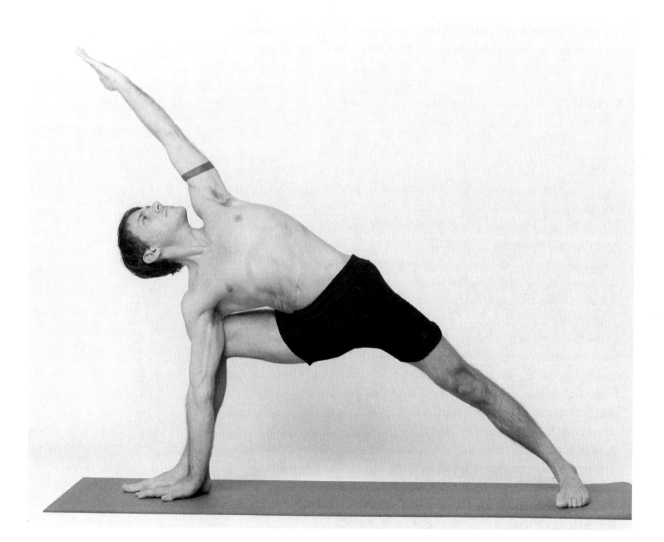

Modifications

- Beginner: If reaching your right hand to the floor is too difficult, an alternative arm position is to bring your right elbow to your right thigh, and then bring your hands together in prayer position in front of your heart. Use the pressing together of your palms to gently leverage the twist. Your left elbow should point straight up.
- Intermediate: From the front, wrap your right arm under your right thigh. Reach your left arm behind your back and clasp both hands together to bind your arms.

Benefits

This pose provides a long stretch for your groins, spine, waist, and shoulders. It also strengthens your legs, knees, and ankles.

Contraindications

Do not do this pose if you have a headache, high or low blood pressure, or insomnia.

Inspiration

A long line of energy is essential in this pose. Imagine creating a line from your back heel through your hip and intercostal muscles, and then up your arm. Once you establish this line, feel yourself breathing into the length of it for a much more buoyant pose. Your hips do not want to sink down with gravity; there is a lightness as both hips lift slightly. When you do not establish that line, gravity wins and the pose becomes much more difficult. Arrive at a state of acceptance, offering only what you can here. Your breath will tell you if you can offer more or if you need to back off a little.

EXTENDED TRIANGLE POSE (UTTHITA TRIKONASANA)

Getting In

- Start in Warrior II Pose (Virabhadrasana II) with your right foot forward.
- Straighten your right leg. Bend from your hips over your right leg, reaching the fingertips of your right hand forward as you shift your torso down. Place your right hand on your right shin or ankle or on the floor to the outside of your right foot. Reach your left arm toward the sky.
- Reaching long through both arms, open your chest. Do not collapse your right rib cage (the side of your rib cage that faces toward the floor). Keep it long. Feel length in both sides of your body.

- Direct your gaze up toward your left hand.
- Breathe deeply. Hold for 5 to 10 breaths or longer.
- To release, rotate and lift your arms and torso back up to Warrior II Pose.
- Repeat on the other side.

Key Actions

- Activate your core to create a lifting sensation up from your bottom hand.

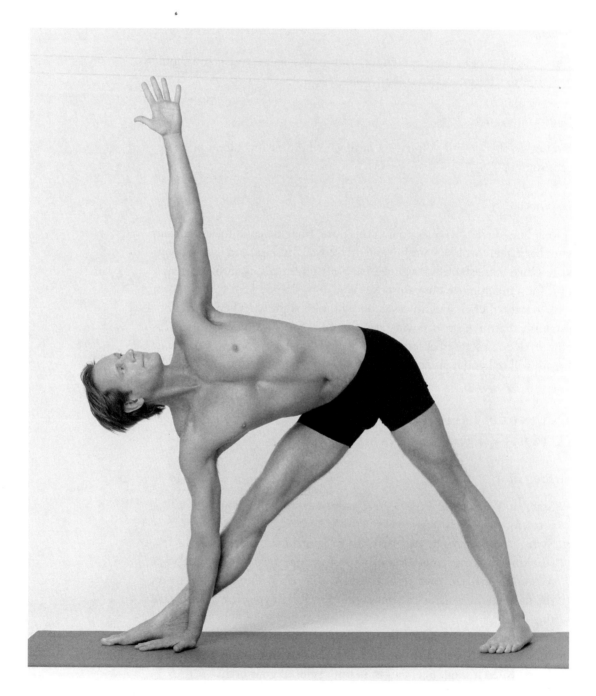

- The position of your feet can be challenging. Make sure to keep the toes of each foot pointed in the direction of that knee. In other words, the toes of your front foot should be facing straight forward. The toes of your back foot are angled in slightly. The openness of your hips will determine the angle of your back knee, which then determines the angle of the back foot.
- Press firmly into the mound of the big toe on your front foot as you focus more of your weight into your back heel. Activate your quadriceps to build more strength in your legs. Your bottom hand should become lighter on your shin or ankle.
- Stack your hips vertically. Lift your top hip and slide the lower hip and sit bone underneath.

Modifications

- Beginner: If looking up does not feel good on your neck, rotate your gaze toward the floor. Instead of lowering your bottom hand way down and gripping your leg, slide your bottom hand a little bit higher up your leg. Think of it this way: the only reason you have your hand there is to prevent yourself from flying away with the energetic lift through your upper arm. Rather than sinking into your bottom arm, use it as the base for that upward lift.
- Beginner: If there is any undue strain on the hamstring of your front leg, soften that knee.
- Intermediate: Deepen the stretch by placing your hand, palm side down, on the floor, inside or outside your front foot.

Benefits

This pose helps you attain a nice stretch in your hips, groins, hamstrings, calves, spine, and shoulders. It also strengthens your thighs, knees, and ankles.

Contraindications

Do not do this pose if you have a headache, high or low blood pressure, or neck issues. If you have high blood pressure, turn your head to look down at your bottom foot.

Inspiration

Give yourself permission to back off in Extended Triangle Pose. Explore greater sensation without trying single-mindedly to get your hand down to the floor. Backing off will give you time to reflect on your form. Is there a breath here that might potentially be healthier? If you find that your spine collapses in the effort to try to reach your foot or the floor, lift up out of the pose a little more. You may find an opening and joy you would not otherwise have experienced.

REVERSE WARRIOR POSE
(VIPARITA VIRABHADRASANA)

Getting In

- Start in Warrior II Pose (Virabhadrasana II) with your right foot forward.
- Your arms are extended out to the sides in a T shape. Turn just your right palm up to the sky, rotating from the shoulder. Drop both shoulders away from your ears. Lower your left arm and rest that hand on the back of your left leg. Raise your right arm toward the sky, with the palm facing behind you toward the back of your mat. Reach through your right arm and the right side of your waist.
- Engage your core and keep your spine straight as you gently bend from your hips, with your torso reaching toward your left leg.
- Direct your gaze up toward your right hand or toward the floor.
- Breathe deeply. Hold for 5 to 10 breaths or longer.

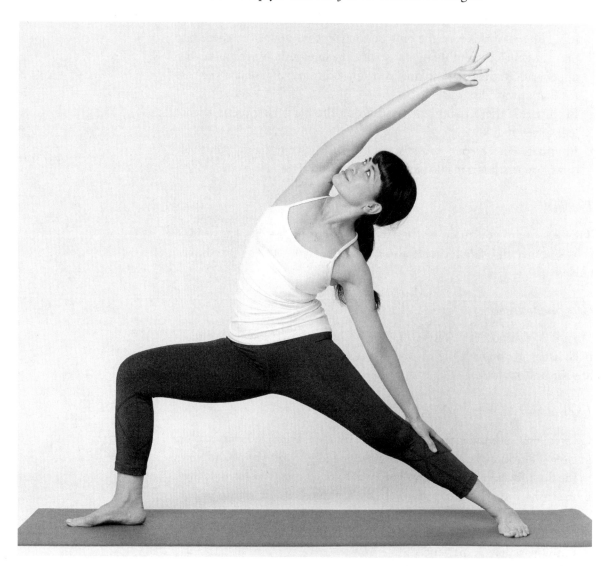

- Release by lifting back up into Warrior II Pose.
- Repeat on the other side.

Key Actions

- When you lean back in this pose, it is easy to abandon what you cannot see: your front knee. Keep your front knee stacked over your heel. The knee tends to collapse inward because of a lack of foundation. Do a visual check at first, then feel and trust it from there.
- Stay strong through your back leg. Do not let the back knee buckle. Keep shooting strength through your entire back leg. Engage your quads and press your back heel away from your torso, lifting through the arch of your back.
- Create space on both sides of your body. With the focus of the stretch on your front side, avoid doing anything weird or crunchy on the other side. If approached in a healthy manner, a nice, long stretch on one side does not need to compromise the other side.

Modifications

- Intermediate: Reach your right arm behind your back and slip your fingers into your left hip crease. Use the fingers of your right hand to coax your left thigh down, creating a deeper bend in your right knee and more opening through the left side of your body.

Benefits

This pose stretches your legs, ankles, hips, groins, and shoulders and strengthens your legs and ankles.

Contraindications

Do not do this pose if you have a backache, neck or back issues, or high blood pressure.

Inspiration

This is a rare lateral stretch that helps to create extension and grace. It often becomes an active rest stop after Warrior II Pose. This pose can be a lot of work, but it feels elegant to bring length into the sides of your torso.

WARRIOR I POSE (VIRABHADRASANA I)

Getting In

- Start in Mountain Pose (Tadasana).
- Inhale and step your left foot behind you about three or four feet, with your heels in a line. In this particular pose, we want the feet as close

to being on one line as possible. However, some students (those who are pregnant or those who have knee concerns) might wish to open the stance a bit wider by walking the front foot out to the side.

- Pivoting on your left heel, turn your left foot out about 45 degrees. Keep your right foot at the top of the mat, with the outer edge of your foot parallel to the outer edge of the mat and the toes facing forward.
- Lengthen your tailbone. Align your spine by stretching up, stacking each vertebra over the other.
- Inhale and extend your arms over your head. Your palms can face each other, about shoulder-width apart, or they can touch.
- Exhale and bend your right knee to a 90-degree angle, aligning your knee over your ankle. Keep your hips forward and squared.

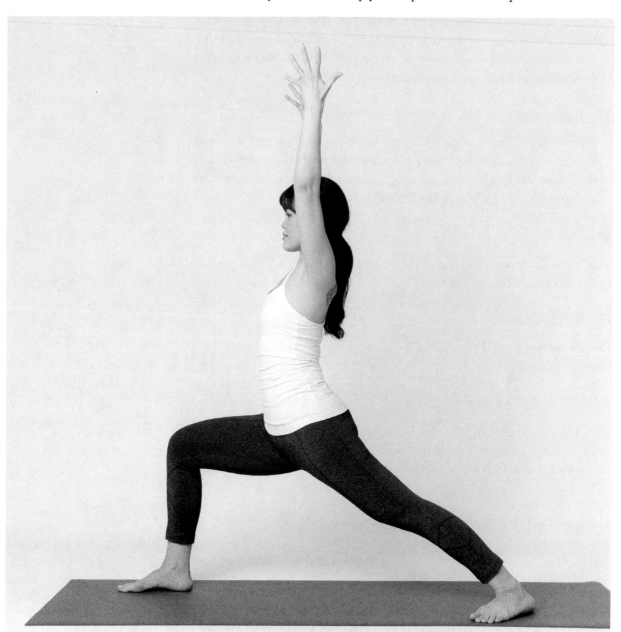

- Draw in your abdominals. Lower your shoulder blades away from your ears and open your chest.
- Send your tailbone and sit bones down to open up your pelvis and hips.
- Direct your gaze forward or up toward your hands.
- Breathe deeply. Hold for 5 to 10 breaths or longer.
- Release by reversing out into Mountain Pose.
- Repeat on the other side.

Key Actions

- Activate your core. Focus on Uddiyana Bandha (Abdominal Lock): draw the place right below your navel in and up while breathing deeply. Feel your tailbone move down slightly. This adjustment alters your breath completely. It brings almost instant relief to any struggle in your lower back.
- Ensure that your hips are squared. The proper alignment will create a sensation of lifting out of your pelvis as well as a feeling of lightness in the pose.
- Your front knee should be in your peripheral line of vision, making it easy to see so you can keep it stacked over your ankle. Make sure it does not collapse in or fall out to the side.

Modifications

- Beginner: To check your weight distribution and balance, lift your front toes. If you are too wobbly, focus on distributing your weight more evenly in both legs. Place more weight on your front heel than on the toes. If you are still struggling with balance, shorten the distance between your feet and walk your front foot out to the side so your feet are staggered about hip-width apart rather than one in front of the other. As your strength and pose improve, lengthen your stance again and bring your feet back in line.

Benefits

This pose improves the balance between your upper and lower body. It also strengthens your back, shoulders, and thighs.

Contraindications

Do not do this pose if you have heart, shoulder, or lower back issues. If you have high blood pressure, modify the pose by bringing your hands to your hips.

Inspiration

When it comes to squaring off our hips, many of us have a mental disconnect. I find I can remedy this simply by reminding myself to square my hips and shoulders. If your back hip is turning toward the back, readjust your stance. Bring your back foot forward a bit and consider turning the foot in more. Focus on trying to build strength in your back leg. You should feel yourself lifting up out of your pelvis, not crunching into your lower back.

WARRIOR II POSE (VIRABHADRASANA II)

Getting In

- Start in Mountain Pose (Tadasana).
- Inhale and step your left foot behind you about three or four feet, with your heels on a line. As in the previous pose, we want the feet as close to being on one line as possible. However, some students (those who are pregnant or those who have knee concerns) might wish to open the stance a bit wider by walking the front foot out to the side.

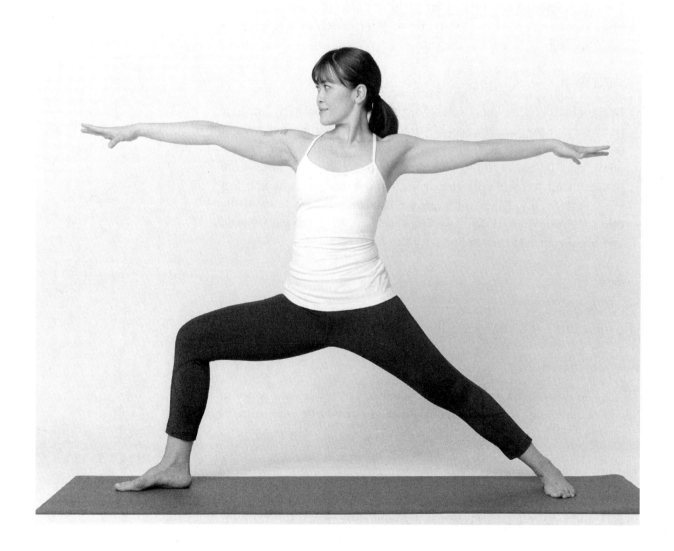

- Keep your right foot at the top of the mat, with the toes pointing straight ahead and the outer edge of your foot parallel to the outer edge of the mat.
- Pivoting on your left heel, rotate your left foot out to between 45 and 60 degrees.
- Open your hips to the left.
- Inhale and extend your arms straight out to your sides, at shoulder height, in a T shape.
- Exhale and bend your right knee to form a 90-degree angle, aligning your knee over your ankle.
- Align your spine by stretching up, stacking each vertebra on top of the other. Maintain a straight spine and avoid letting your torso lunge forward over your right knee. Stack your shoulders over your hips. Slide your shoulders down, away from your ears.
- Deepen the stretch and let your hips drop. Lower your sit bones and tailbone. Contract your thighs to maintain support and lengthen the horizontal stretch.
- Direct your gaze just beyond your right middle finger.
- Breathe deeply. Hold for 5 to 10 breaths or longer.
- Release to Mountain Pose.
- Repeat on the other side.

Key Actions

- Create a wide base. Open your stance by sliding your left foot farther back and making the top of your right thigh more parallel to the floor.
- Make sure your shoulders are over your hips and not leaning forward. Your arms and hands should be extended out to the sides, over your feet. Stretch from the fingertips of one hand to the fingertips of the other.
- Make a connection between your inner right knee and your upper right pelvic bone, along with the whole groin area. Feel the tripod of your pelvis and sit bones open wide.
- Try tapping into Uddiyana Bandha (Abdominal Lock) in this manner: Move one hand to your lower back and encourage your tailbone to drop. Place your other hand below your navel. As you gently tilt your tailbone down, encourage the place just below your navel to move in and up. Notice the difference when you manually activate Uddiyana Bandha. It opens your breath to the full capacity of your lungs.

Modifications

- Beginner: If your balance is wobbly, move your feet about hip-width apart so they are staggered rather than in line.
- Beginner: Eventually, your front thigh should be parallel to the floor. At first, however, it's okay if the thigh is not quite parallel and your stance is slightly closer together. You'll get there.

Benefits

This pose stretches your legs, ankles, hips, groins, and shoulders and strengthens your legs and ankles.

Contraindications

Do not do this pose if you have a backache or neck or back issues. If you have high blood pressure, modify the pose by bringing your hands to your hips.

Inspiration

In this pose, there is a tendency to look around. The average student will focus on anything in the room other than being in the pose; the same is true for Monkey Pose (Hanumanasana). But the irony is that this pose becomes even more challenging if you are looking for an escape to take you out of the experience. The time you spend in this pose may seem like an eternity, but it is typically only five short breaths. Trust your breath, commit to your *drishti*, and flow safely through the experience. If you are finding it too easy, change it up—widen your stance a little and drop deeper into the pose.

CHAPTER 10

Standing Balance Poses

THESE POSES can really help us out when we are stressed or feeling scattered. Try them earlier in your practice before you get fatigued; it may help to use a wall if you are having a tough time. Positioning your arms out to the sides can help as well. In all balance poses, keeping your eyes open and focused makes a big difference.

It's easy to get frustrated with these poses. After all, it's hard enough to balance on two feet sometimes! Remember, you are asking one leg to do all the work, which requires a lot of lower body focus and mental concentration. This is a good place to work on dealing with life's little frustrations. Being patient and persistent is key. A standing balance practice will reward you with increased coordination and attention.

This is also a great place to practice falling, which is an important lesson in life. We need to fall down a few times so we can learn how to get back up.

HALF-MOON POSE (ARDHA CHANDRASANA)

Getting In

- Start in Extended Triangle Pose (Utthita Trikonasana; page 107) with your right foot forward.
- Place your left hand on your left hip. Bend your right knee and place your right hand on the floor about 12 to 24 inches in front of your foot. Exhale and straighten your right knee while lifting your left leg until it is parallel to the floor. Flex your left foot. Stack your left hip on top of your right hip.

- Lift your left arm toward the sky with the palm facing away from your body. Simultaneously rotate your head and torso until your gaze is straight up to the sky over your left shoulder.
- Stretch your arms in opposite directions and feel the horizontal stretch in your torso and spine.
- Breathe deeply. Hold for 5 to 10 breaths or longer.
- Release into Mountain Pose (Tadasana). Move into Extended Triangle Pose on the left side and repeat.

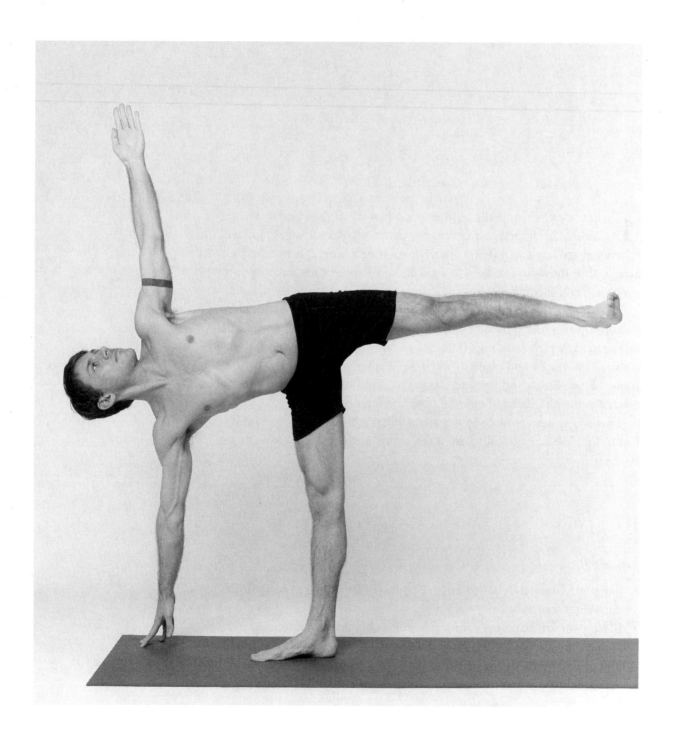

Key Actions

- If the knee of your standing leg is unstable, you should address this first. Remember, always start with a safe foundation and proper alignment. Your front foot is parallel to the outer edge of your mat, with your front knee stacked over the ankle and hip stacked over hip. In stacking poses, make sure you build the foundation from the bottom up. If your hips are not stacked and both legs are not working in harmony, the upper leg becomes dead weight—and it is harder to lift dead weight.
- *Drishti* is important, but a *drishti* that is comfortable for one person may not be comfortable for another. Instead of getting caught up in trying to look skyward, notice if your neck is comfortable. If it feels better for you, look to the side or even down. It does not necessarily matter *where* you look, but *how* you look. Try and focus on something with softness, and let that bring some stillness to the pose.
- A lot is going on in this pose, so it is important to check in and be sure you are not creating more tension or struggle. Always breathe first.
- A bonus: This pose works your medial glutes (the muscles on the outer sides of your pelvis), which do not get to work in a lot of poses.
- Do create a strong foundation, whether it is with your legs, arms, or core.

Modifications

- Beginner: If you are having trouble reaching the floor with your hand, bend your standing knee and/or use a block under your hand.
- Intermediate: Play with lifting your bottom hand a few inches off the floor and using your core muscles—not your hand—to support your weight.

Benefits

This simple sideways bend has a powerful punch. It stretches your shoulders, groins, hamstrings, thighs, and calves and strengthens your spine, abdomen, buttocks, and thighs.

Contraindications

Do not do this pose if you have low blood pressure, a headache, or insomnia.

Inspiration

Patanjali, the author of the Yoga Sutras, would have greatly appreciated Half-Moon Pose. There is a softness here that creates a sweet lightness. If you overwork the pose without allowing that lightness and those long lines of energy to occur, you miss out. When a strong foundation is created, a lightness happens. In certain poses, if you go deeper into the pose, it actually becomes easier. This is one of those poses.

Eagle Pose (Garudasana)

Getting In

- Start in Mountain Pose (Tadasana).
- Begin to balance your body by evenly pressing all parts of your feet into the floor and finding your center. Focus on your navel.
- Bend your right knee, shifting your weight to your right foot.
- Lift your left leg and cross your left thigh over the right. Wrap your left ankle behind your right calf. Hook the toes of your left foot so the left big toe rests on the lower inside of your right calf.
- Deepen the bend in your right knee, sitting down into your buttocks.
- To realign your posture, tuck your tailbone, pressing your pelvis forward slightly and drawing your abdominal muscles in. Keep your spine straight.
- Now extend both arms out to the sides with your palms open and facing down. Bring your arms together and cross your right arm over your left, joining them at the elbows.
- Bend both arms up so your fingers are pointing toward the sky. Wrap your forearms to bring your palms together. (The palms won't align; you will likely have the fingers of one hand against the palm of the other.)
- Lift your upper arms so they are parallel to the floor at shoulder height. Draw your shoulders down and away from your ears.
- Press your intertwined forearms away from your face until they are perpendicular with the floor.
- Breathe deeply. Feel the stretch in your shoulder blades, thighs, quads, and glutes.
- Hold for 5 to 10 breaths or longer.
- Release into Mountain Pose. Repeat on the other side.

Key Actions

- Different yoga schools teach the arm position differently. Some say "arms up," like I've described above, while others say, "squeeze arms down," so the elbows move close to the chest. I like to play with both positions. The different variations work different parts of the arms and shoulders and require varying amounts of strength and flexibility.
- When you carefully stack your bones and bring your body into alignment, Eagle Pose requires less endurance, and your body can begin to relax into the pose.

Modifications

- Beginner: If intertwining your legs and arms is difficult initially, start by simply placing your left ankle over your bent right knee, creating a 90-degree angle with your left knee. Cross your right arm over your left, taking hold of the opposite elbows. Hold 5 to 10 breaths. Release and repeat on the other side. If you have trouble with balance, use a wall for support. Stand with the wall behind you, and let your flat spine slide slowly down the wall.

- Beginner: If you can't seem to get your palms to meet, aim for any part of your hands joining, even lacing your fingers. Rotate the wrists so that the pinky sides of the hands face forward. A little patience and persistence goes a long way here!

- Intermediate: Hinge forward from your hips, bring your elbows beyond your top knee, and fold your torso forward so it is hugging your top thigh.

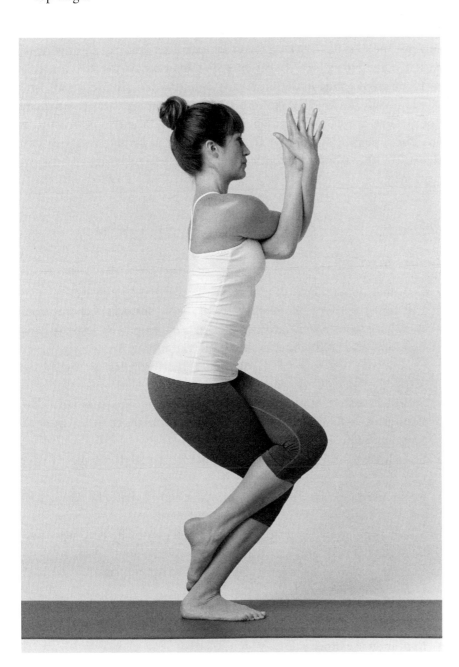

Benefits

This limb-twister gives a good stretch to your hips, thighs, shoulders, and back and strengthens your ankles and calves. When everything is in alignment, it also releases tension in your shoulders.

Contraindications

Do not do this pose if you have arm, shoulder, hip, or knee issues.

Inspiration

Everything we do on the mat is related to what we do off the mat. We think, *If I find balance on the mat, maybe I can find balance off the mat.* Try to imagine the specifics. Back off for a moment. See if you can allow yourself to stay in the pose a little longer by easing up or modifying it.

If you are sweating in this pose, the sweat from your elbows should land right on your top knee. Make sure your knees and hips are centered and your elbows are stacked right above your knees. If the arm positioning is too distracting, bring your hands to your hips and gently press your hips down. Use the strength of your core to feel your chest lifting up.

LORD OF THE DANCE POSE (NATARAJASANA)

Getting In

- Start in Mountain Pose (Tadasana).
- Lift your right foot back and up toward your buttocks, bending your right knee to get there. Reach your right arm behind you with the hand open and take hold of the inside of your right foot.
- Square your hips forward. Gently reach your right leg up toward the sky, as though your toes were reaching over your head.
- Simultaneously extend your left arm forward with the palm facing the floor (or take Chin Mudra by touching the forefinger to the thumb). Splay your fingers.
- Strengthen your core. Grow your spine tall through the top of your crown.
- Press your raised foot backward into your right hand. The strength of your leg helps to open your shoulder and chest.
- Slowly begin to fold your torso forward so it eventually becomes parallel to the floor. Do not let your spine collapse; it should arch.
- Feel the stretch in the hamstrings and thighs of both legs.
- Direct your gaze forward.
- Breathe deeply. Hold for 5 to 10 breaths or longer.
- Release back into Mountain Pose.
- Repeat on the other side.

Key Actions

- This is one of my favorite poses. Everything is going on: a nice back-bend, a great hamstring stretch, a little core maintenance. Don't be surprised if one side feels dramatically different from the other.
- From the beginning, the placement of your standing leg is important. The standing leg remains really active throughout the pose. Make sure your foundation is set by stacking your joints properly.

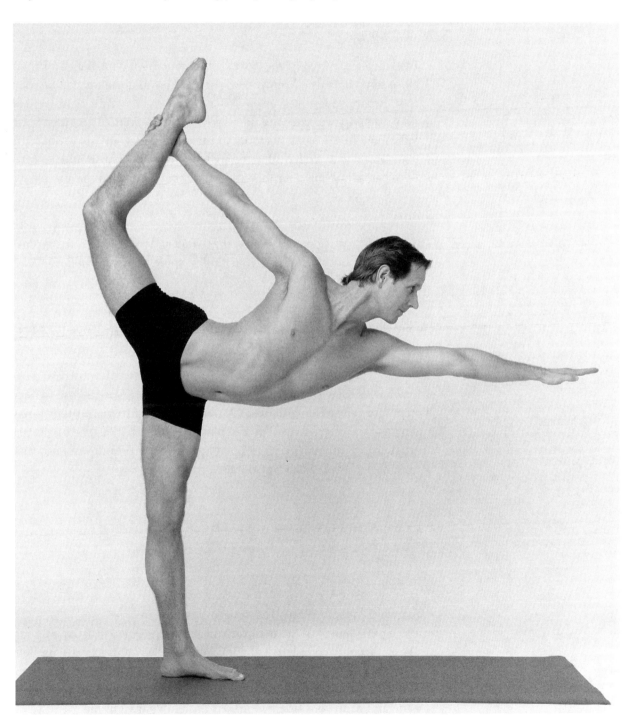

- Before taking your back leg up, allow your knees to "kiss," which keeps your bent knee from splaying too far out to the side. Make sure you have the proper grip with your hand. Then, as you lift your back leg, hug both legs toward the midline.
- One way to make sure you have the proper handhold on your foot is to check that your thumb and big toe are close to each other. Holding your foot correctly will help your hips stay in proper alignment and let your shoulders open nicely.

Modifications

- Intermediate: Once in the pose, bring your right foot high and then close to your body. Wrap your right hand around the outside of your foot. Rotate your elbow up and over your shoulder. Your right hand is now reaching over your shoulder with the elbow pointed up. Align your left elbow in the same position and take hold of your right foot with your left hand as well. Both arms are reaching over your shoulders, with both hands holding your foot and lifting up to lengthen the stretch.

Benefits

This pose is a real opener. It stretches your abdominals, thighs, groins, and shoulders and strengthens your thighs, spine, hips, and ankles.

Contraindications

Do not do this pose if you have back issues or high or low blood pressure.

Inspiration

A lot of folks love to open their hips in Lord of the Dance Pose (which is often also called Dancer's Pose), but it's important to master the closed hip in this traditional asana. You can play around with it; just be conscious of what you're doing. Own the opening and do it on purpose, not just because you are being lazy or not paying attention.

EXTENDED HAND TO BIG TOE POSE (UTTHITA HASTA PADANGUSTHASANA) VARIATION

Getting In

- Start in Mountain Pose (Tadasana).
- Place your hands on your hips or in prayer position in front of your chest. Ground your left leg. Find strength by contracting your left thigh to help root your leg into the floor. Square your hips to the front.
- Lift your right knee toward the sky. Reach for your foot with your right hand and wrap your first two fingers around your right big toe.

- Holding onto the toe, flex your foot and straighten your right leg until it is mostly parallel to the floor.
- Keep your right shoulder drawn back so your shoulders remain squared to the front of the mat. Straighten your leg only to the extent that you can keep your shoulder back. Keep your shoulders and hips stable and aligned.
- Support everything in this pose by igniting your core. Lengthen your tailbone down and let your pelvis establish a base for your core. Extend your spine and neck.

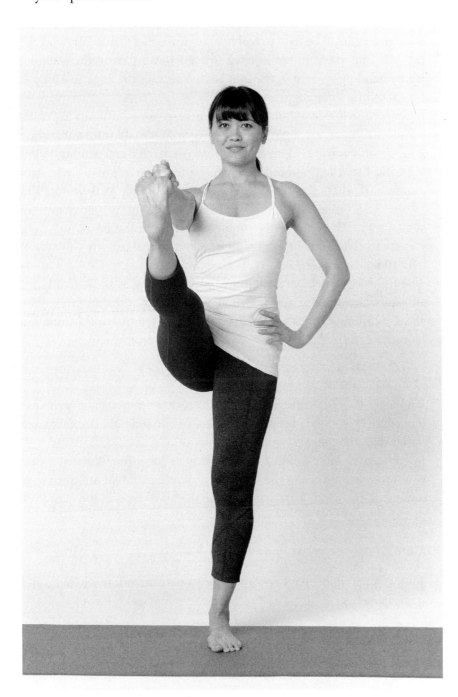

- Keep your left hand on your left hip or in half-prayer position in front of your heart.
- Direct your gaze forward.
- Hold for 5 to 10 breaths or longer.
- To release, exhale and release your foot, returning to Mountain Pose.
- Repeat on the other side.

Key Actions

- In this pose, students become excited about getting the top leg straight and extended, but for me, it is more about straightening and extending the standing leg. We tend to feel happier if we stay focused on what we can see. But when we really safeguard the lower part of the standing leg by building an arch in the foot and protecting the knee and hips, it brings us into safer alignment.
- Extend your upper leg only if you can keep your standing leg completely strong and straight. Do not take your shoulder forward when you extend your leg. Many students do not have the flexibility to extend the lifted leg without collapsing their spine. This is a perfect example of when you should be wary of becoming goal-oriented in a pose. It is important to remember that it is never about getting somewhere; it is about being honest and having integrity about where you are in this moment in this pose. Allow your flexibility to develop over time.
- The front leg may be extended at hip level as long as the standing leg and spine are straight and the shoulders remain down the back. (We all have different limbs and torsos of differing lengths, but I think the objective can still be the same—a solid foundation.)

Modifications

- Beginner: If your hamstrings are tight, use a strap around your extended foot, or simply keep your top knee bent and hold the bent knee rather than the toe.
- Intermediate: After holding the initial pose for a few breaths, rotate your extended leg out to the side. Keep your leg straight and your hips squared to the front. Turn your head to the opposite side and gaze over that shoulder.

Benefits

As long as your spine stays straight, any stretch in your arms, legs, and ankles is beneficial. This pose also strengthens the backs of your legs.

Contraindications

Do not do this pose if you have ankle or lower back issues.

Inspiration

Build the foundation for this from the bottom up. When you "cheat," you set yourself up to disconnect from your breath and the ultimate aim of the practice. Struggling with your breath does not make the pose any easier. To paraphrase Patanjali: keep it strong, keep it stable, be cool. There should be an element of comfort and (dare I say it?) joy in every pose. If it is just about the bulldog mentality of doing it "right," the end result will be unrealistic expectations that will only make you tighter in the long run.

TREE POSE (VRKSASANA)

Getting In

- Start in Mountain Pose (Tadasana).
- Inhale and shift your weight onto your left foot.
- Bend your right knee. Draw the knee up to hip level, so you are balancing on your left foot.
- With your right hand, take hold of your right ankle, and place the sole of your foot against the inner thigh of your left leg, with the toes pointing down.
- Extend your arms straight out to your sides, palms facing forward, on a slight diagonal from your body.
- Bring your hands into prayer position in front of your heart.
- Either leave the hands in prayer position or, if you prefer, raise the arms overhead, keeping the palms together or letting them come apart to any comfortable distance. If your arms are raised, stretch up through your fingertips.
- Stretch down through your sit bones.
- Focus your gaze on a point in front of you that is not moving, or up toward your hands.
- Breathe deeply. Hold for 5 to 10 breaths or longer.
- Release back into Mountain Pose.
- Repeat on the other side.

Key Actions

- As your foot presses into your thigh, let the thigh press back a little.
- Activate your core and lengthen your tailbone down. Minimize the sway in your lower back to reach taller.

Modifications

- Beginner: Instead of immediately opening my knee to the side, I bring my knee up to center first and then allow it to open to the side like a hinge. This feels safer for the hip and knee joints. If your hips are uneven, bring your bent knee slightly forward. If you struggle with balance, place your foot lower on your standing leg, where it can help you stabilize. This may be as low as the inner calf, ankle, or even with your toes resting lightly on the floor. *Never* place your foot against your knee or push your knee outward.

Benefits

This pose stretches your groins, inner thighs, chest, and shoulders; improves your balance; and strengthens your thighs, calves, and groins.

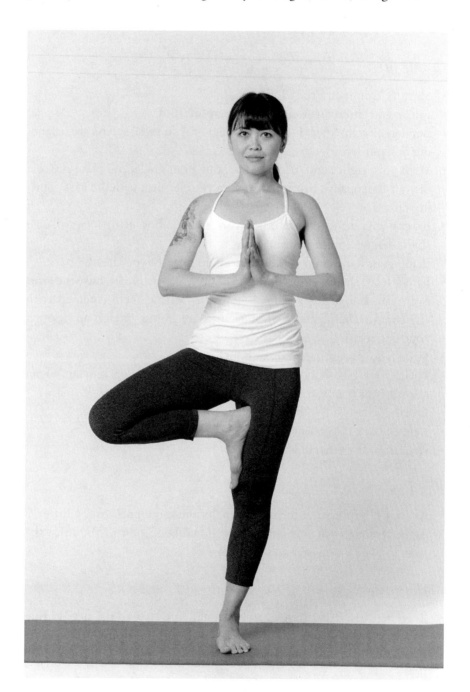

Contraindications

Do not do this pose if you have a headache, insomnia, or high or low blood pressure.

Inspiration

This is a wonderful pose for beginners, because you can find so much delight in the balance alone. There is something splendid in the simplicity of Tree Pose, that feeling of instant gratification when you realize you can stand on one foot. There is also something beautiful about impersonating a tree. If you are having issues with balance, repeat these words to yourself: "I am grounded." Focus on the roots moving out of your feet and into the earth as you extend your gratitude to the sky. You are rooted and blossoming at the same time. How cool is that?

CHAPTER 11

Core

MANY YOGA ENTHUSIASTS don't like to take core work seriously. When building strength in our legs with lunges and Warrior Pose (Virabhadrasana) or working on our upper body with Four-Limbed Staff Pose (Chaturanga Dandasana) and arm-balancing poses, we cannot neglect the reality that our center is what keeps it all together. Core work is often considered aesthetic when, in fact, the core initiates everything we do. It's not about getting six-pack abs. I like to work my core because it helps guarantee the stability and safety of the rest of my foundation. Developing your core will bring a greater sense of ease and lightness to all of your yoga asanas. Besides, anything we do with present-mind awareness is a yogic practice in itself.

BICYCLE

Getting In

- Lie on your back with knees bent.
- With your head resting on the mat, clasp your hands behind your head.
- Raise your legs 10 to 12 inches off the floor and imitate a pedaling action: Bend one knee up toward your torso and straighten the opposite leg. In a fluid motion, bend the straight leg while straightening the bent knee and pressing away with the extended heel.
- Now add your head, chest, and shoulders. Lift them off the mat and allow the weight of your head to drop into your clasped hands as you move from side to side.
- As you pedal, reach an elbow toward the opposite knee, alternating elbows and always initiating the movement from the strength of your core.

- Breathe deeply in concert with your movements for about 30 to 60 seconds.
- To release, lower your legs.

Key Actions

- Move from your core and ensure that your elbows remain nice and wide.
- Avoid stretching your neck forward. There should be no strain on your neck; the weight of your head rests in your clasped hands.

Modifications

- Beginner: If this pose is too intense, rest your head on the mat, bring your hands under your buttocks, and pedal your legs. This variation can help you avoid low back strain.
- Intermediate: Play with the height of your legs, taking them lower or higher. Notice any difference you feel in your body and where you are getting the best workout. Explore the position of your feet by flexing and then pointing your toes to see which one gives you a unique challenge.

Benefits

Like a real bicycle ride, this pose develops core strength and provides a nice stretch for your legs.

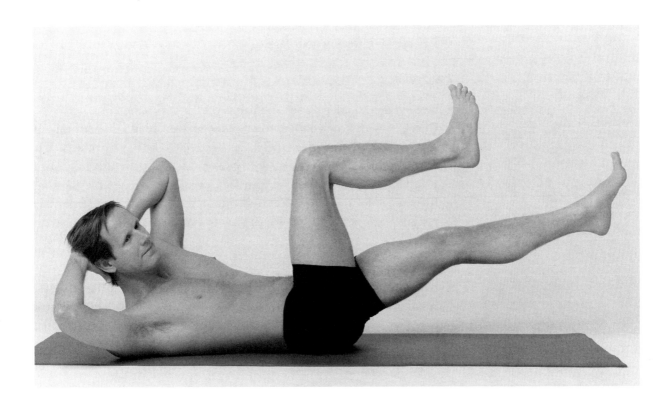

Contraindications

Do not do this pose if you have back issues.

Inspiration

Be aware of your level of engagement in this pose. Are you simply pedaling fast without really feeling anything? Or are you breathing in sequence with your movements and staying present and connected?

REVOLVED ABDOMEN POSE (JATHARA PARIVARTANASANA)

Getting In

- Lie on your back with your legs straight and both arms out to the sides in a T shape and palms on the floor.
- Lift your legs straight up toward the sky.
- With control, lower your legs to the left, parallel to your outstretched arm, until your feet hover a few inches from the floor. Turn your head and gaze to the right. Keep your legs straight and your feet flexed. Hold for 3 breaths.
- Lift your legs back up to the sky. With control, lower them to the right, and turn your gaze to the left. Hold for 3 breaths.
- Repeat three times on each side. Activate your inner thigh muscles to keep your legs together.
- Your gaze alternates from side to side.
- Release by lowering your legs.

Key Actions

- Keep your shoulder blades and palms pressing into the floor.
- Check in with how you feel to see how far you should go with this. If it is too much work to keep your legs extended, bend your knees. If it is uncomfortable for your neck to gaze in the opposite direction, turn your head to the same side as your legs, or keep it in a neutral position. If you need to touch your feet to the floor, move with caution from this resting place as you lift your legs back to vertical.

Modifications

- Beginner: Lie on your back with your arms in a T shape. Lift your legs, bending your knees in toward your body with your legs together, until your shins are parallel to the floor. Keeping your arms in the T shape, rotate from your hips and take your legs from one side to the other. Let your outer knee touch the floor, then rotate back to the other side, and repeat. Don't let your knees rest on the floor; find the core strength to simply touch them lightly.

- Intermediate: In this fluid version of the pose, your legs imitate the motion of a windshield wiper. With both legs extended to the sky, let your left leg fall to the left (parallel to your arms) and hover above the ground without touching. Let your right leg follow but at a distance of 10 to 12 inches. Hold for 3 breaths. Swing your right leg up and over to the right side, letting the left leg follow. Alternate from side to side.

Benefits

Adjust this pose to your comfort level to get a good core-strengthening workout. This pose also aids digestion and elimination.

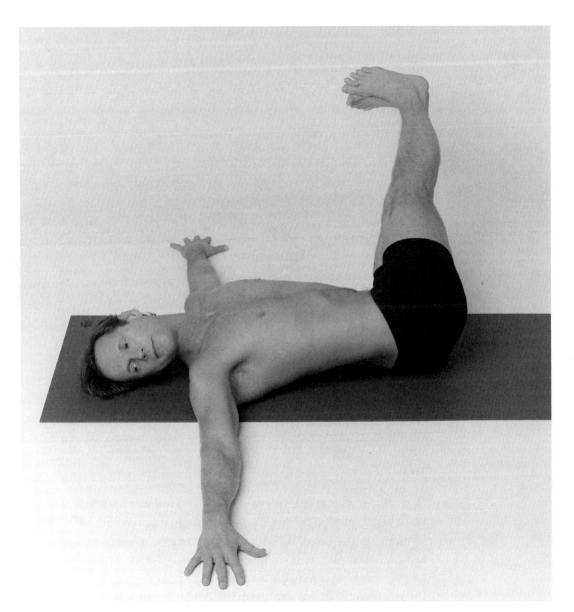

Contraindications

Do not do this pose if you have back issues.

Inspiration

Come to this pose with courage, not fear. Courage builds confidence, and confidence builds strength. A brave heart will help you move your body carefully and thoughtfully through each pose. Remember, the most important thing in yoga is always moving in harmony with the breath. If your breath is labored, try something different and make any necessary changes to allow your breath to return to a deeper, more rhythmic state.

LEG LIFTS

Getting In

- Lie on your back with your legs out straight and your hands, palms down, at your sides. Slide your hands under your buttocks, and touch your thumbs.
- With your head on the mat, elongate your neck and draw your shoulders away from your ears.
- Inhale as you activate your abdominal muscles. Raise your legs straight up toward the sky, perpendicular to the floor.
- Exhale and slowly lower your legs until they are about a foot off the mat.
- Hold for several breaths or longer.
- Inhale and raise your legs back up.
- Remember to breathe deeply.
- Repeat the lifts a few times.
- To come out, bring your knees to your chest and release your lower back.

Key Actions

- Imagine your lower black flattening and your navel drawing toward the floor.

Modifications

- Beginner: If your abdominals are weak or your lower back feels stressed, place your hands on the floor, palms down, beside your buttocks instead of tucked under them. If you are overarching your lower back, lift your legs higher or play with your range of motion—or bend your knees and let your heels tap the mat when you lower your legs.
- Intermediate: If there is no strain in your lower back, lift your head and upper shoulders while maintaining the action of your navel drawing

down to the floor. Exhale as you lower one leg to the ground. Inhale as you raise it back up. Alternate legs.

- Advanced: With both legs pointed up toward the sky, bend one knee and place the ankle on the opposite thigh just below the knee. Lower and raise your legs in this position. Alternate legs.

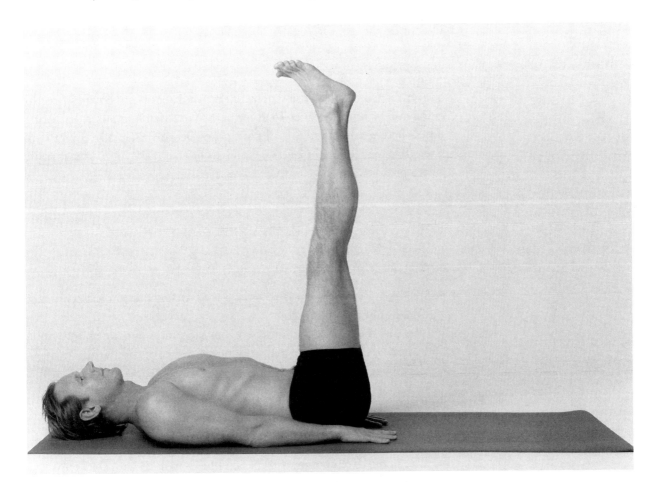

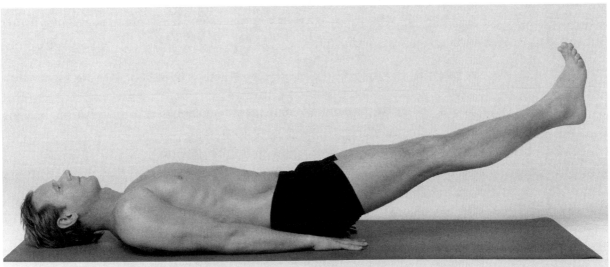

Benefits

While strengthening your core and back and toning your abdominal muscles, leg lifts also relieve lower back pain.

Contraindications

Do not do this pose if you have back issues.

Inspiration

Everything comes from the center. Energy radiates up and down, strengthening and bringing balance to every part of us. Standing poses, balancing poses, backbends—they are all core poses because they all require core strength and stability. In fact, we could argue that *every* yoga asana is really a core pose.

FULL BOAT POSE (PARIPURNA NAVASANA)

Getting In

- Start in Staff Pose (Dandasana; page 196), sitting upright with your legs straight out in front of you.
- Inhale as you lean back slightly on your sacrum, balancing on the tripod created by your tailbone and sit bones. Keep your spine straight.
- Place your hands, palms down, behind your buttocks, or slip your fingers under your thighs.
- Exhale.
    Pose 1: Lean farther back onto your sacrum and lift your legs. Bend your knees toward your chest until your shins are parallel to the floor. Extend your arms parallel to your shins with the palms facing each other.
    Pose 2: Engage your core and extend one leg until your foot is higher than your head. Retract the leg. Extend the opposite leg. Keep alternating.
    Pose 3: Extend both legs together until your feet are higher than your head.
- In each variation, gently draw your shoulders back and down, opening your chest and lifting your heart.
- Hold each variation for 30 seconds or more.
- Direct your gaze forward.
- To come out, lower your feet to the floor.

Key Actions

- Notice what happens with your spine when you straighten one leg. Does your weight go back to your tailbone? By noticing your weight distribution, you become more responsible for the fuller expression of the pose. Then it is a much more honest and raw awakening.

- This pose really works your core. I think of the core as a corset around the torso, wrapping all the way around the lower back from the rib cage to the knees. It's important to make sure we apply equal work to the areas of our body that aren't easily in view, the core included! It is essential to remember to keep your core engaged, your shoulders down, and your chest lifted.

Modifications

- Beginner: Start with your legs bent at a 90-degree angle, heels level with your knees. Straightening one leg up at a time, notice what happens to your back, your shoulders, and your foundation.
- Intermediate: Move between Poses 1, 2, and 3, according to your comfort level. Shaking can be a sign of tight hip flexors, a tight lower back, or misalignment in your spine. If you are shaking on the leg extensions, return to the first pose. Try again. Hold for a shorter time as you build your strength.

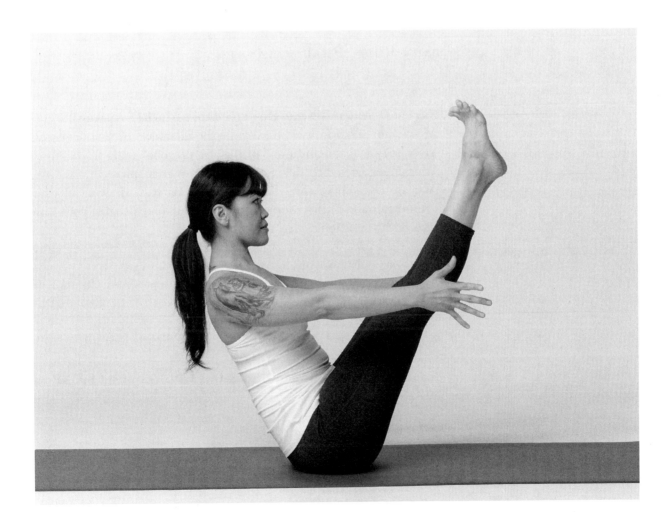

Benefits

This full stretch strengthens your core, stimulates your internal organs, improves digestion, stretches your hamstrings, and tones the muscles of your lower back.

Contraindications

Do not do this pose if you have diarrhea, a headache, low blood pressure, heart issues, insomnia, or lower back issues, or if you are pregnant or menstruating.

Inspiration

Being the boat can be much more fun than being *in* the boat. Like a maiden voyage, start slowly. Discover the mechanics of this pose, and feel the nuances and subtleties of being a boat. It may be easier to do crunches and Leg Lifts, but Full Boat Pose is honest-to-goodness core work. Many people avoid this pose because, when it is done right, it is really hard. It is tempting to give up. But what's the point of that? Try and do this pose with humility: if you roll onto your back, just giggle and start again.

PLANK POSE (PHALAKASANA)

Getting In

- Start in Downward-Facing Dog Pose (Adho Mukha Svanasana).
- Move your torso forward until your shoulders are over your wrists. Your body will slide into one plane, at a diagonal angle to the floor. Your upper arms should be perpendicular to your spine.
- Activate your upper core. Lengthen the stretch by drawing in your abdominals and lifting your sit bones and tailbone, keeping your hips level with your shoulders.
- Press the backs of your thighs up toward the sky, push your heels away from you, and allow your heart center to move forward.
- Spread your shoulder blades wide across your upper back. Do not collapse your spine.
- Relax your neck, face, and throat muscles.
- Breathe deeply, and direct your gaze down or slightly forward.
- Hold for 5 to 10 breaths or longer.
- Release back into Downward-Facing Dog Pose, or rest in Child's Pose (Balasana).

Key Actions

- Avoid sagging your hips too low or lifting them higher than your shoulders. Create a lightness in your hips with the support of your core and legs.

- If you feel yourself sagging in the middle, press your palms into the floor and draw in your abdomen.
- Keep your arms straight and strong; stacking your arm joints—wrists, elbows, shoulders—makes this pose easier on your arms than you might think.
- Try not to lock your elbows.

Modifications

- Beginner: To build up core strength, start in a kneeling version of Plank Pose. From Table Pose (on your hands and knees), lean into your arms and press your palms into the floor. Slide your knees back about 12 inches, lengthening your torso according to your comfort. Draw in your abdominal muscles to be sure you keep your spine from collapsing.
- Intermediate: Lower into Four-Limbed Staff Pose (Chaturanga Dandasana).

Benefits

Welcome to core-conditioning boot camp! This pose also strengthens your arms, wrists, and thighs.

Contraindications

Do not do this pose if you have carpal tunnel syndrome.

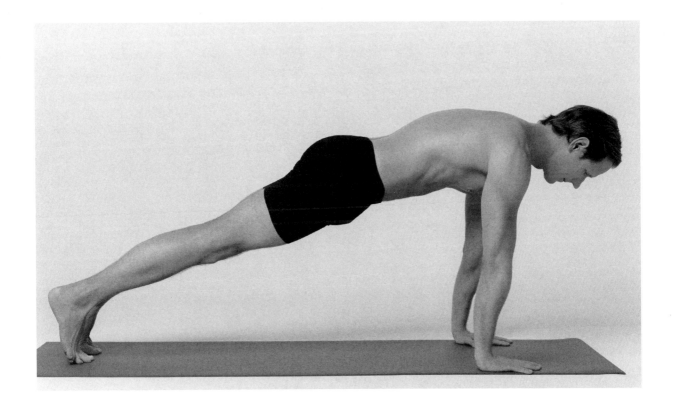

Inspiration

Plank Pose is about endurance; staying with it helps develop strength and lessen reactivity. Any part of your body that is not participating or actively engaged is like dead weight that puts unnecessary stress on your joints. By strengthening and engaging your entire body, you create support that will allow you to lift up and out of your joints, relieving stress and compression. A half asana (being only partially in the pose) can be more harmful and challenging than a full pose.

CHAPTER 12

Arm Balances

ARM BALANCES have many of the same benefits as standing balance poses, but much of the work is shifted to the upper body and core. A healthy imagination and mental discipline is essential. Of course, flexibility in the shoulders, spine, and hip flexors will be of great help. Think of these poses as sculptures. Take your time warming up with preparatory poses like Plank Pose (Phalakasana), Garland Pose (Malasana—a simple, low-seated squat with the feet comfortably apart and the toes turned out in the direction of the knees), and even Full Boat Pose (Paripurna Navasana). These will prepare the core and other support muscles.

EIGHT-ANGLE POSE (ASTAVAKRASANA)

Getting In

- Start in Staff Pose (Dandasana; page 196), sitting upright with your legs straight out in front of you.
- Draw your right knee toward your chest with your foot off the ground, so your right thigh is perpendicular to the floor and your right shin is parallel to it.
- Reach your right arm under your right knee and, using your hands if necessary, tuck your right shoulder under your right knee.
- Place your hands flat on the floor on either side of your hips. Your left leg remains extended forward, and your right leg remains lifted over your right shoulder.
- Shift your weight onto your hands and lift your buttocks and legs off the mat as you straighten your arms. Your left leg and right shin should be parallel.

- Now draw your legs together and place your left ankle on top of your right foot.
- Bend your elbows while you fold your torso forward from your hips toward your feet.
- Twist your hips and legs to the right.
- Continue lowering your torso and head until your head is in line with your feet.
- Squeeze your thighs toward each other. Press out through the balls of your feet.
- Direct your gaze forward or down at the floor.
- Breathe deeply. Hold for several breaths or longer.
- To come out, release your legs and straighten your arms while rolling onto your buttocks. Come back to Staff Pose.
- Repeat on the other side.

Key Actions

- Make the pose look and feel effortless, not as though you are holding on for dear life. To strengthen the pose through your core and legs, squeeze your bound upper arm with your inner thighs.
- This is a balancing pose! Keep it steady. Remember that your navel, or center, is between your hips. If you start rocking your hips back and forth, you are likely to tip over.

Modifications

- Beginner: Build up to Eight-Angle Pose by starting on your buttocks with your hands on the floor. Bend your right leg over your right shoulder and cross your left ankle over your right. Your legs can be extended or your knees bent.

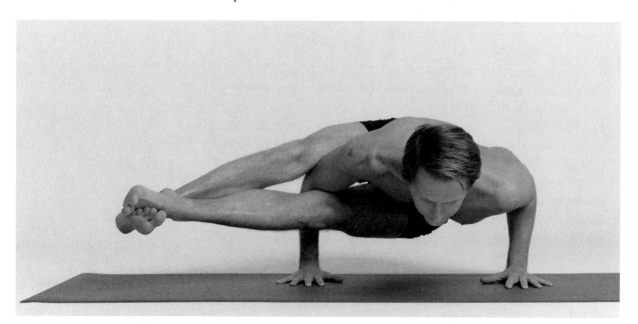

Benefits

This pose strengthens your wrists, arms, and abdominals. Also called the Eight Bend Balance, this is an opportunity to get in touch with your yogic center of balance.

Contraindications

Do not do this pose if you have shoulder, wrist, or lower back issues.

Inspiration

The concept of your center of gravity as the center of your weight distribution is easy to grasp in most yoga poses. For example, as you lift one leg in Tree Pose (Vrksasana), you can easily compensate by shifting your weight to your other (standing) leg. In arm balances, however, you may feel like a contortionist as you do your best to find your center. When your limbs are no longer evenly balanced alongside your body, finding your center of gravity can be disorienting. To master this balancing act, it is important to take a holistic view of the pose and notice each contraction and extension. Determine which muscles you need to use to support the lightness and balance of this pose. Then relax the others. That way, you won't waste energy where it's not essential.

CROW/CRANE POSE (BAKASANA)

Getting In

- Start in Garland Pose (Malasana, or a deep squat). Bring your hands to prayer position in front of your chest. Turn your toes out about 45 degrees, and press your heels into the floor.
- Begin to shift your torso forward, straighten your arms, and place your palms on the floor in front of you, shoulder-width apart. Splay your fingers and ground your palms.
- Place your knees as high up on the backs of your upper arms as possible. Do not let your elbows splay out; squeeze your upper arms toward parallel.
- Exhale. Lifting onto the tips of your toes, continue to shift your torso forward, and move your shins onto your upper arms.
- Transferring your weight onto your arms and hands, lift your buttocks higher. Your torso should move toward parallel to the ground.
- Lift your feet off the floor. Draw your big toes together.
- Hug your inner thighs in toward the midline.
- Direct your gaze forward to the floor out in front of your fingertips.
- Breathe deeply. Hold for 5 to 10 breaths or longer.
- To release, press your hands into the floor and lower your feet and torso back into Garland Pose.

Key Actions

- This is another beautiful balancing pose. There is only you, your center, and gravity. Focus on finding balance in each movement and the overall pose.

Modifications

- Beginner: To build up to the pose from Garland Pose, gradually transfer more and more weight onto your arms. Rock back and forth, allowing your feet to lift and lower as you work on building your strength, about 5 to 10 breaths as you are able.
- Intermediate: Extend one leg behind you in a straight plane with your torso. Breathe deeply for about 5 to 10 breaths. Alternate legs.

Benefits

Once you have found your balance, you will enjoy a more lengthy stretch through your spine and neck. This pose also strengthens your arms and core.

Contraindications

Do not do this pose if you have wrist issues or are pregnant.

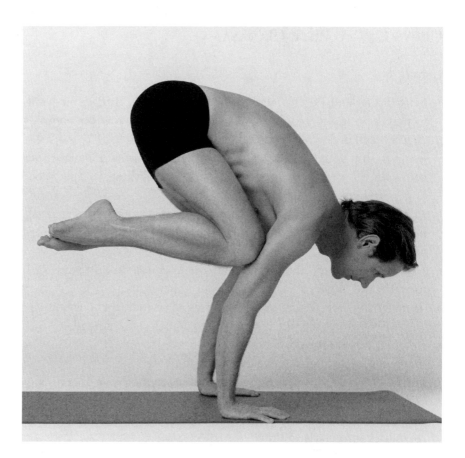

Inspiration

Moving in and out of Crow/Crane Pose is a good opportunity to get in touch with your core, including your pelvis and spine. Many poses start by tucking the tailbone to start moving the pelvis and spine into alignment. Focus on bringing your core into alignment by lengthening your lower back and moving your tailbone down before going into Crow/Crane Pose. You now have a strong plane, rather than a disjointed torso, to balance on your hands.

SHOULDER-PRESSING POSE (BHUJAPIDASANA)

Getting In

- Start in Garland Pose (Malasana, or a deep squat). Bring your hands to prayer position in front of your chest. Turn your toes out about 45 degrees, and press your heels into the floor.
- Begin to shift your torso forward, placing your palms on the floor about hip-width apart. Lift your sit bones toward the sky until your thighs are near parallel to the floor. Splay your fingers and ground your palms.
- Tuck your right upper arm under your right thigh, just behind the knee. Your right palm is now flat on the ground, slightly behind you. Repeat on the left side.

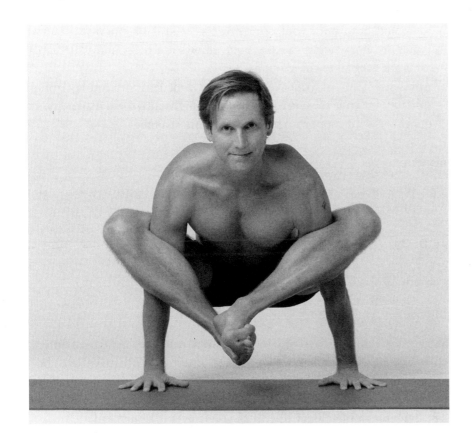

- Rock your weight onto your hands. Strengthen and straighten your arms by pressing your hands into the floor. Focus on centering your navel as you lift your hips. Lift your feet and legs off the ground.
- Squeeze your legs toward each other and cross your left ankle over your right. Keep your legs active. Press out through the balls of your feet.
- Direct your gaze forward.
- Breathe deeply. Hold for 5 to 10 breaths or longer.
- To come out, release your ankles, bend your knees, and return to Garland Pose.
- Repeat the pose with your right ankle crossed over your left.

Key Actions

- This pose provides another wonderful example of strength and grace. To strengthen the pose, squeeze your upper arms with your thighs while solidifying your core and legs. Draw your navel center up and in.
- A nice rounding of the back is required in this pose. Do not try to keep your spine straight. Think about opening up your vertebrae from behind.
- Activate Uddiyana Bandha (Abdominal Lock) and Mula Bandha (Root Lock).

Modifications

- Intermediate: Roll with it. Balancing between your arms, shift your torso and head until your crown or forehead is on the mat. Your sit bones are now facing the sky, your elbows are bent, and your upper arms are parallel to the ground.
- Advanced: Unhook your feet and widen your legs into full horizontal splits. Point your toes. Press your inner thighs into the outside of your upper arms for support. This is a real groin stretcher.

Benefits

This pose uses your center of gravity as a supporting force while you strengthen your arms, wrists, and shoulders.

Contraindications

Do not do this pose if you have wrist issues or are pregnant.

Inspiration

Most of us think of our belly button as our center of balance. Did you know that you actually have two centers of gravity? The navel area balances the legs and torso, while a second center of gravity in the head balances the head and spine. So where should you focus your balance? Try drawing an imaginary line from your navel to your head.

Four-Limbed Staff Pose
(Chaturanga Dandasana)

Getting In

- Start in Downward-Facing Dog Pose (Adho Mukha Svanasana) and move into Plank Pose (Phalakasana).
- Shift the weight of your torso forward onto your arms.
- Tuck your tailbone and lengthen your spine. Keep your chest and shoulders broad as you hug your shoulder blades into your back ribs.
- Bend your elbows to move lower and forward until your upper arms and body are parallel to the floor. Keep your elbows and upper arms alongside your torso, with your elbows lined up over your wrists.
- Brace the position. Press the balls of your feet and your hands into the floor for support. Draw in your abdominals, and strengthen your thighs.
- Direct your gaze out in front of your fingertips to keep your neck long and your shoulders back and down.
- Breathe deeply. (This pose, when done correctly, can help build upper body strength, especially if you stay in it for 5 to 10 breaths. Otherwise, this is a connecting pose in the vinyasa practice that is traditionally entered into with an exhalation and exited with an inhalation.)
- To release, press your hands into the floor and lift your sit bones toward the sky, coming back into Downward-Facing Dog Pose.

Key Actions

- This pose may look uninteresting, but the truth is it's a great abdominal workout. Your abdominals keep your hips from sagging by maintaining

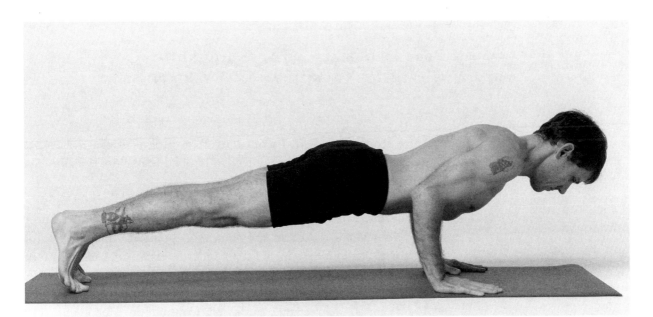

a level line from hips to shoulders. To avoid collapsing in the middle, work your abdominals. Inhale. Tuck your tailbone and feel your chest opening.

- Note how this nice stretch through your abdominals and chest is compromised if you hunch your shoulders, which causes your chest to draw in.

Modifications

- Intermediate: Raise your head so your gaze is forward and lift higher onto the tips of your toes. To avoid placing too much weight on your toes, contract your abdominals and hamstrings for support. Shift more weight to your upper torso and arms.
- Advanced: Lift one leg toward the sky as high as is comfortable. Release and alternate legs.

Benefits

This pose is prized for its abdominal workout. It also strengthens your arms, chest, and wrists.

Contraindications

Do not do this pose if you have lower back, shoulder, or wrist issues.

Inspiration

Focusing on your center of gravity without connecting it to deep breathing is like trying to ride a bicycle with flat tires. Breathing not only helps us to be present in the moment but also invites more stability in the core, making it easier to bring everything into alignment.

POSE DEDICATED TO SAGE KOUNDINYA (EKA PADA KOUNDINYASANA) VARIATIONS

Getting In

- Move from Downward-Facing Dog Pose (Adho Mukha Svanasana) to Plank Pose (Phalakasana) to Four-Limbed Staff Pose (Chaturanga Dandasana).
- There are two variations of this pose:
  Variation 1: Bring your right leg forward so the thigh is hooked over your upper right arm and your leg is pointing straight forward, with the foot flexed, but the toes may be extended. Line your foot up with your head.
  Variation 2: Bring your right leg under your left leg until the right leg is at a 45-degree angle to the left. Continue to extend your right

leg to the left, with toes pointed forward. Keep both legs straight, with your outer right thigh braced on your upper left arm.

- Bend your elbows as you bring your weight forward, allowing your left foot to lift off the ground. Maintain the lift in your upper body so your chest is parallel to the floor as well.
- For support, activate your core. Stretch the toes of both feet, lengthening your legs, stretching your groins, and finding balance for your torso.
- Gaze is either down or to the side.

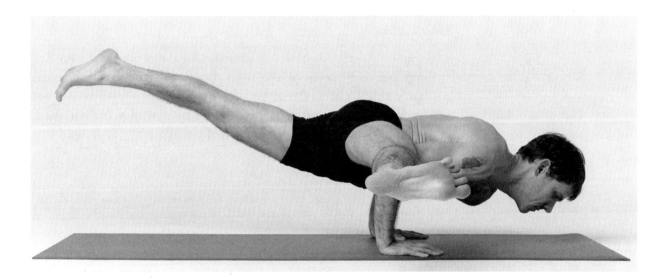

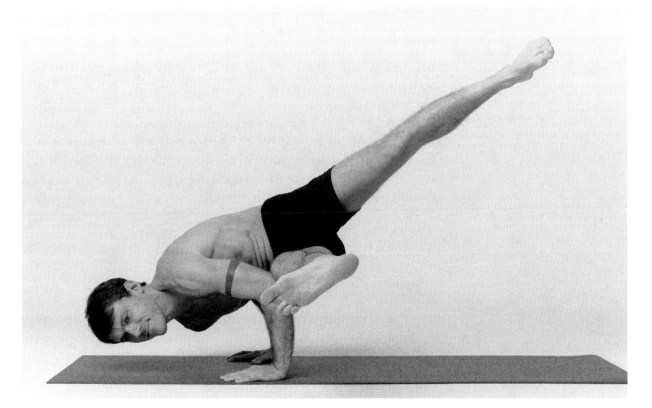

- Breathe deeply. Hold for 5 to 10 breaths or longer.
- To come out, release your legs and press back into Downward-Facing Dog Pose.
- Repeat on the other side.

Key Actions

- Your arms are providing support, but they are not a centering mechanism. Instead, your center of gravity is in your core; engaged abdominal and back muscles are the key to levitation in this pose.

Modifications

- Beginner: Rest the foot of your extended leg on its side on the floor.
- Intermediate: Place more weight on your arms. Then create a steeper slope with the plane of your body by lifting your back leg higher and lowering your torso while maintaining lift and openness in your chest.
- Advanced: Straighten one leg in front of you and the other behind you.

Benefits

This near-split is a great groin stretch. It also strengthens your abdominals, arms, and wrists.

Contraindications

Do not do this pose if you have lower back, shoulder, or wrist issues.

Inspiration

Your neck is an extension of your spine, so there are many reasons why you want to focus on elongating it. First and foremost, it is necessary to preventing neck injury. Second, it is part of your alignment and balancing act. Achieving a single plane with your torso and head helps create a greater sense of ease in your poses. Third, consider the weight your neck carries. Many of us hang our head over our computer and desk all day, placing unnecessary stress on our bodies. Keep your neck strong and long and your head balanced whenever possible.

FLYING CROW POSE (EKA PADA GALAVASANA)

Getting In

- Start in Tree Pose (Vrksasana) with your left foot on the inside of your right thigh.
- Move your left foot from inside your right thigh to just above your right kneecap. Slide your left ankle just beyond your right thigh and flex your foot.

- Bend your right knee slightly and fold your torso forward until your hands are touching the ground in front of you, shoulder-width apart.
- Hook your left ankle under your right armpit and really catch your right tricep with the toes of your left foot by strongly flexing that foot. The top of your left foot is now against your upper right arm.
- Place your palms flat on the floor.
- Lift your hips until your spine is roughly parallel to the ground.
- Shift your weight forward onto your hands.
- Hug your upper arms toward each other.
- Raise your right foot up toward the sky until it forms a plane with your torso. Extend out through the ball of your right foot.
- Direct your gaze downward.
- Breathe deeply. Hold for 5 to 10 breaths or longer.
- To come out, lower your right foot, release your left leg, and jump both legs straight back to Plank Pose. From here, move into Downward-Facing Dog Pose (Adho Mukha Svanasana) and back to Tree Pose to repeat on the other side.

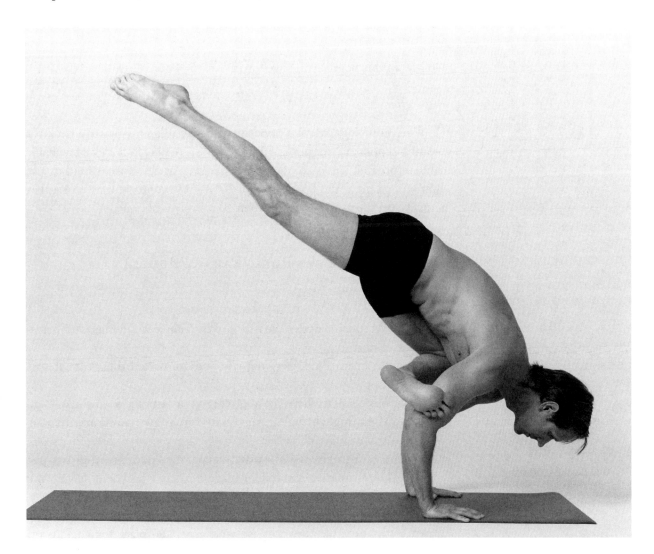

Key Actions

- Be sure your navel is always at the center of this pose. There are not many opportunities to fidget with balance here if you don't get it right. If you remain centered, you will float effortlessly into the pose.
- Handstand (Adho Mukha Vrksasana) can help you build strength for this pose. Beginners can explore using the wall for support in Handstand while developing arm and core strength.

Modifications

- Beginner: Build up to this pose through Crow/Crane Pose (Bakasana). Draw your knees high up onto your arms, close to your shoulders. Point your feet and sit bones toward the sky.

Benefits

This pose strengthens your abdominals, arms, and wrists. It also helps with centering and balance.

Contraindications

Do not do this pose if you have lower back or wrist issues.

Inspiration

Hooking your leg over the opposite arm like a latch is a nifty trick for creating support in this pose. While this posture may look more mechanical than organic, looks are deceiving. The key to this pose is fluidity and awareness. Often, the poses that look the most contorted are those that actually feel the most balanced when your body is aligned.

SIDE CROW/CRANE POSE (PARSVA BAKASANA)

Getting In

- Start in Mountain Pose (Tadasana) with your feet together and hands in prayer position.
- Bend your knees and lower your sit bones until your thighs are almost parallel to the floor.
- Twist your torso to the right and place your left elbow on the outside of your right thigh, bringing your hands into prayer position with your gaze over your right shoulder.
- Squeeze your thighs together, and keep your knees pointing straight ahead. Draw your right shoulder blade into your back and deepen the twist.
- Bend your knees farther to lower your sit bones to within an inch or two of the ground. Now, release your arms and place your hands on

the floor to the right of your legs, palms down. Your fingers should be splayed and facing away from you, with your hands shoulder-width apart. Place your right hand about 2 to 3 feet away from, and in line with, your right hip. Your left arm should be touching the outside of your right thigh.

- Shift your weight onto your hands, allowing your torso and sit bones to rise.
- Let your legs lift while straightening them out to the side.
- Hug your upper arms toward each other to keep your elbows from splaying.
- Keep your legs together and elevated parallel to the floor, as your right leg rests on your upper left arm and elbow. Flex your feet.
- Direct your gaze slightly forward of your fingertips.
- Breathe deeply. Hold for 5 to 10 breaths or longer.
- To come out, release your feet to the floor and reverse out of the pose, coming back into Mountain Pose.
- Repeat on the other side.

Key Actions

- Hanging out in this pose is easier than you might think if you have found your center of gravity. From the first moment that you begin to twist, let your navel lead you. However heavy your legs may seem, stay focused on your center of gravity. With the proper balance, and by stacking your elbows over your wrists, your legs will feel lighter.
- If you honor the technique, moving into the pose step-by-step, the outer strength of the pose will serve as a reliable foundation. If you jump into the posture haphazardly, chances are something will be misaligned.

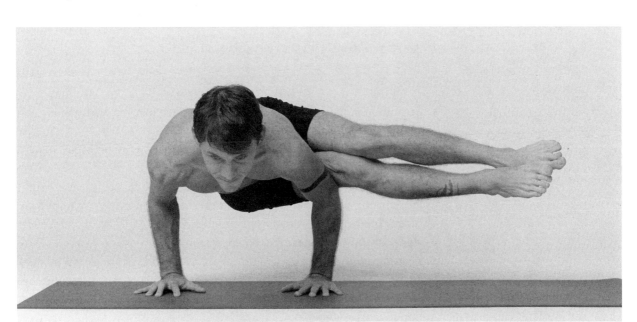

Modifications

- Beginner: Build up to the pose by extending your legs to the side but keeping your feet grounded on the mat.
- Intermediate: Straighten your arms or your legs. Your lower leg will remain slightly bent and hooked over your elbow.

Benefits

Although your body appears to be in suspended animation in this pose, it is not possible to defy gravity. Your abdominals, arms, and wrists are strengthening as they work hard to keep you suspended. You can also master centering in this pose.

Contraindications

Do not do this pose if you have lower back or wrist issues.

Inspiration

One of the primary goals of Bhakti Yoga is the complete surrender of self. Sometimes this is mistakenly interpreted as an excuse for letting it all hang loose—like in Corpse Pose (Savasana). However, this isn't possible in arm balances, because letting anything hang loose would quickly cause you to lose your balance and fall over. Consider moving away from any greedy or ambitious thoughts about "conquering" a certain pose, and instead free your mind to focus on the balance and harmony inherent in that pose. Allow yourself to discover its subtleties and the experience of being in it. The pose is not about finding balance by fighting gravity. There should be no "fight." It is about being aware and attuned to the natural balance in gravity.

FIREFLY POSE (TITTIBHASANA)

Getting In

- Start in Mountain Pose (Tadasana) with your feet hip-width apart and your arms at your sides.
- Fold forward, hinging from your hips and raising your sit bones toward the sky. Bend your knees slightly.
- Wrap your right arm between your legs and then behind your right leg, so your right hand is placed flat on the mat outside your right foot. Simultaneously, tuck your right shoulder behind your right knee. Keep this position and repeat it on the left side.
- Shifting your weight onto your arms and hands, start lowering your sit bones toward the floor. Straighten your arms and lift your legs off the ground. Use your lower thighs and upper calves to hug your upper arms.

- Continue to straighten your arms, lifting your sit bones higher, while straightening your legs as you press out through the balls of your feet.
- Keep your spine straight. Imagine a puppet string from the crown of your head, lifting you up through each vertebra.
- Direct your gaze forward.
- Breathe deeply. Hold for 5 to 10 breaths or longer.
- To come out, release your legs and reverse out into Mountain Pose.

Key Actions

- Loosen up! While straightening your legs, you will feel the action in your hamstrings. If your hamstrings are tight, consider practicing poses to loosen them, such as Reclining Big Toe Pose (same as Big Toe Pose, but performed lying on the floor, face up), Head-to-Knee Forward Bend (Janu Sirsasana), or Happy Baby Pose (Ananda Balasana).
- This is another pose in which you want to look and feel as if you are floating effortlessly. Really activate your core and find your center of gravity. Think of your core as an invisible block that is keeping you propped up. Your tailbone, pelvis, and spine are working together to create strength and support.
- Your legs really have to work here too. Otherwise, they will lose out to gravity. Contract your quadriceps, lengthen your hamstrings, and stretch a straight line from your sit bones to your toes, energetically extending your toes forward.

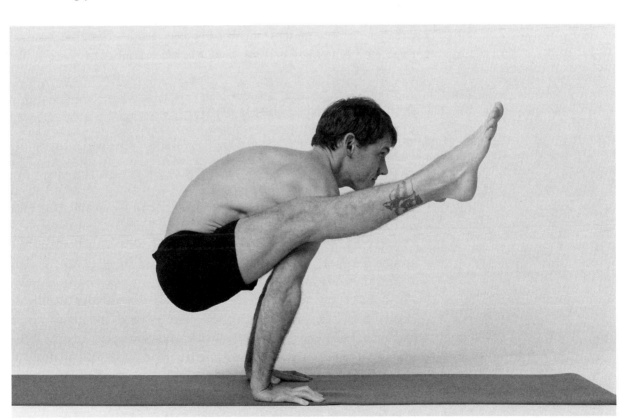

Modifications

- Beginner: If you are not ready to lift your legs, touch your toes together on the floor in front of your head. Your legs will form a triangle.
- Intermediate: Rock your hips and sit bones forward until they are facing front. Simultaneously, pivot your legs up and reach your toes toward the sky.

Benefits

When you achieve grace in the pose, it becomes effortless and easy to build strength in your arms, shoulders, and wrists. It also stretches your hamstrings.

Contraindications

Do not do this pose if you have lower back or wrist issues or are pregnant.

Inspiration

Firefly Pose is a nice, graceful pose in which to explore alignment of your spine. In this pose, we can see strength and grace work together. At first glance, it looks like your arm muscles are working overtime to defy gravity and keep your body hovering above the floor. But your arms cannot do this job alone. The real strength in the pose comes from the grace in your spine. It is through the proper alignment of your spine that you find real support and balance. Muscles, no doubt, can help provide support in a pose, but the pose must be anchored by your center of gravity. You will not find your center and balance in your muscles alone.

SIDE PLANK POSE (VASISTHASANA)

Getting In

- Start in Plank Pose (Phalakasana).
- Shift your weight to your left arm.
- Rotate your torso and hips open to the right, letting your right leg stack on top of your left leg. You will be resting on your left hand and the top of your left foot. Reach your right arm toward the sky. Anchor your left arm on the floor, with your left shoulder stacked directly over your left wrist. Rotate your torso in the direction of the sky.
- Align your body on one narrow plane. Tuck your tailbone slightly to engage your core, direct your pelvis gently forward, and draw in your abdomen. Lengthen your spine and elongate your neck.
- Press your left hand into the floor and lengthen the stretch up through your right hand, opening your chest.
- Squeeze your inner legs together, stretching from your toes through your thighs and hamstrings.

- Direct your gaze toward the sky. If this is uncomfortable for your neck, look down or straight ahead.
- Breathe deeply. Hold for 5 to 10 breaths or longer.
- To come out, return to Plank Pose. To relax, recline in Child's Pose (Balasana).
- Repeat on the other side.

Key Actions

- It is important to get your alignment right. The hand on the floor should be lined up with the heel on the floor. Your body forms an upward sloping line. Your arm joints should stack on top of each other.

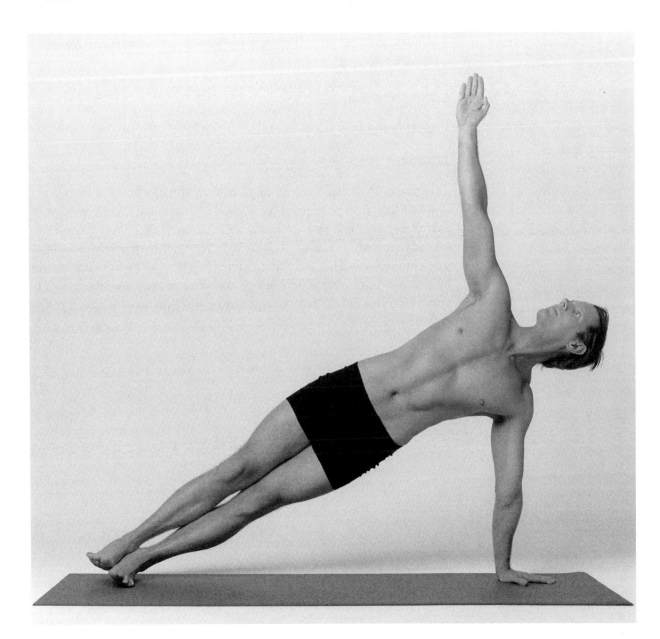

Modifications

- Beginner: For more support or to take the pressure off your wrist, place the forearm of your grounded arm flat on the floor with your elbow directly under your shoulder. Or for a good hip stretch and an alternative sense of balance, bend your top knee and place your foot flat on the floor in front of your bottom knee.
- Intermediate: Extend your upper leg straight up toward the sky and take hold of your foot or big toe with your extended hand. Ground down through your hand on the floor to strengthen your foundation. Start to rotate the sole of your grounded foot toward the floor, so it eventually presses flat.

Benefits

This pose gives all your limbs a good stretch and strengthens your abdominals, arms, legs, and wrists.

Contraindications

Do not do this pose if you have shoulder or wrist issues.

Inspiration

Take the time to explore your alignment in all yoga poses. The straight slope in this side pose provides a good opportunity to fine-tune your overall alignment. If you are in the habit of carrying a heavy bag on one side of your body, for example, you might feel added stress from misalignment in your shoulder and spine. Something may feel a little off in your hips as you stack your legs. Once you've assessed any misalignments in your body, you can do extra strengthening work on the side that is out of balance.

CHAPTER 13

Inversions

INVERSIONS CAN CHANGE our perspective about almost everything. Technically, an inversion is a pose in which the heart is situated higher than the head. Seeing the world from this new point of view can bring a great deal of instantaneous personal growth. We can become much more reasonable and forgiving when we see things in such a different way.

Inversions also counteract the normal gravitational pull on the body. Because of this, they are said to help relieve back pain and aid the function of the cardiovascular system (by creating more efficient blood flow to the heart and increased blood flow to the head); the endocrine system (by stimulating the pituitary, thyroid, and parathyroid glands); and the nervous system (through a possible increase in cerebral spinal fluid, which flows from the brain to the spinal cord).

They also help many of us grow fearless and brave as we gently make friends with the idea of flipping ourselves upside down.

HANDSTAND (ADHO MUKHA VRKSASANA)

I'm a strong believer in learning Adho Mukha Vrksasana against a wall, so this is how I teach it. Once you have the foundation, you'll get to experience the joy of a free-floating upside-down-world away from the support.

Getting In

- Start in Downward-Facing Dog Pose (Adho Mukha Svansana) with your hands approximately 8 inches away from the wall and shoulder-width apart, palms flat on the floor.
- Direct your gaze toward your hands.

- Step your right foot forward about halfway.
- Bend your right knee, and kick your left leg straight up. Let your right leg follow, so your legs are parallel to the wall.
- Bend your knees and place the soles of both feet against the wall. Or let your heels or legs touch the wall for more support and balance.
- If and when you are ready, activate your core and legs and lift your body away from the wall.
- To deepen the stretch and strengthen the pose, press your hands into the floor. Draw your abdominals in toward your spine and your sit bones and tailbone toward your feet in the air. Lengthen the stretch up through your torso, legs, and toes. Press your elbows straight.
- Keep your gaze straight down, between your hands.
- Breathe deeply. Hold for 3 breaths or longer.
- To come out, drop one foot to the floor, with control, and then the other.

Key Actions

- Turning our body upside down can turn our sense of perspective upside down too. Sometimes we even lose our ability to reason for a breath or two. This can be a good thing for those of us who tend to get "stuck in our heads," but if you feel disoriented, calmly return your awareness to your breath. Keep your gaze steady and feel your ability to reason return.
- Whether you are receiving support from the wall or a trustworthy friend, or going it on your own, be sure to really activate your hands, wrists, and forearms, strengthening through your arms. Let your inner guide repeat, "strong arms, strong arms, strong arms."
- Keep your legs active and pay particular attention to engaging and lifting your inner thighs. Become more aware of your pelvis and the connection between your lower and upper extremities by activating your core.
- Begin to tap into the sensation of lifting from your core. Instead of using momentum to "kick" into Headstand, use the power of your abdominal muscles to maneuver your legs into the air. Go slowly, and notice how your core is the true power behind this pose.

Modifications

- Beginner: You can build your confidence and core strength by using the wall a different way: Come into Downward-Facing Dog Pose with your heels touching the wall where it meets the floor. Walk your legs up the wall until they create a 90-degree angle with your body. Press your hands into the floor, elongating your neck and spine. As you brace yourself against the wall, keep your gaze between your hands, and begin to orient yourself to being upside down. You can really have fun with this pose. Here are a few variations:

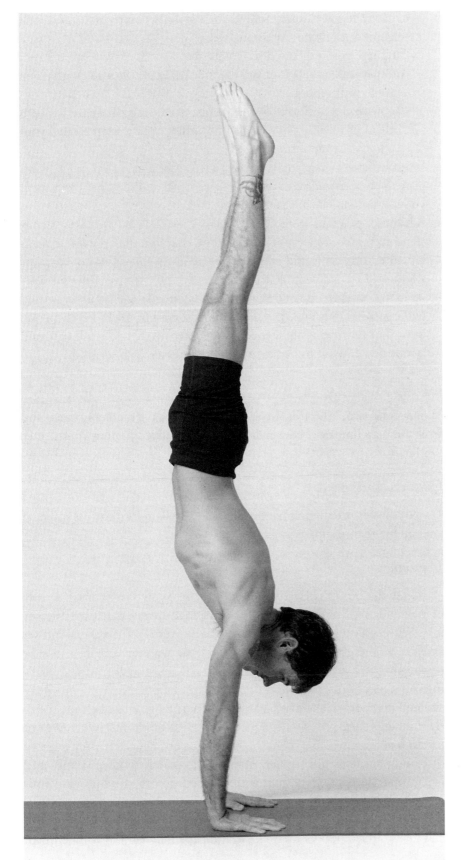

Lift one leg at a time, hold as long as feels comfortable, and then come back down. Alternate legs.

Alternate pointing and flexing your feet.

Alternate taking one foot and then the other off the wall, working up to no wall support.

Play with the position of your hands, narrowing the space between them or turning your hands outward. Or put a strap around your elbows for support.

- Intermediate: When you are ready, instead of kicking up, actively engage the lower *bandhas* to lift your legs. Try it and see what happens. If you fall, you do not have far to go.
- Advanced: Starting from Crow/Crane Pose (Bakasana) makes Handstand even more of a challenge. Lift one knee and then the other, making sure your arms and shoulder girdle are stable. Try not to allow side-to-side movement or wobbling in your pelvis; this causes instability in the pose. Keep your elbows stacked directly over your wrists and build up to Handstand. If you decide you are not ready for this pose, instead of just giving up and collapsing, decide that you will try again tomorrow. Allow it to be fun, and try not to take it so seriously.

Benefits

When done properly, this pose strengthens your shoulders, arms, and wrists. It also improves your balance as you practice finding your center of gravity.

Contraindications

Do not do this pose if you have high blood pressure or heart issues, or if you are pregnant or menstruating.

Inspiration

It is often the fear of falling that keeps us from trying inversions. So many of the students I am blessed to serve have already decided whether or not they can do Handstand before they even start. When this mind-set takes hold, the grace of a beginner is lost. So whether you are a new or seasoned yogi, I suggest coming to this pose as a beginner so you are willing to let go of your preconceptions and see the practice as a gift. Many students approach Handstand with the attitude that it must be conquered. By thinking of the pose as a conquest, a collapse might feel like the fall of the Roman Empire, magnifying your feelings of defeat. If your mastery of Handstand does not happen right away, commit to keep trying until it happens. Be gentle and kind with yourself. Focus on improving your technique and mentally reward yourself with every attempt. Experts say that it takes ten thousand tries to become good at something! Start today and give yourself permission to be in it for the long haul. It will be worth the effort.

Plow Pose (Halasana)

Like Shoulderstand (Salamba Sarvangasana), Plow is a powerful pose, but it can be harmful if you enter it mindlessly and skip over the basic foundational points.

Getting In

- Start in Shoulderstand (page 167)
- Gently lengthen your neck and draw your shoulders away from your ears.
- Depending on how much support you need, you have a few options for hand position:
    Place your hands on your hips for support.
    Place your arms on the floor behind your back, with palms down for leverage.
    Interlock your hands behind your back.
- Bending at the hip joints, lower your straight legs over your head until your toes are resting on the ground behind your line of vision. Flex your feet so the soles are facing away from you.
- If your toes do not touch the floor, or if you need more support, place your hands on your lower back.
- Draw your chin away from your chest to lengthen your neck and relax your throat and tongue.
- Direct your gaze up toward your navel.
- Breathe deeply. Hold for 5 to 10 breaths or longer.
- Coming out of this pose is a good abdominal workout. Lower your buttocks to the floor, then use your abdominal muscles to lower your legs slowly to the floor.

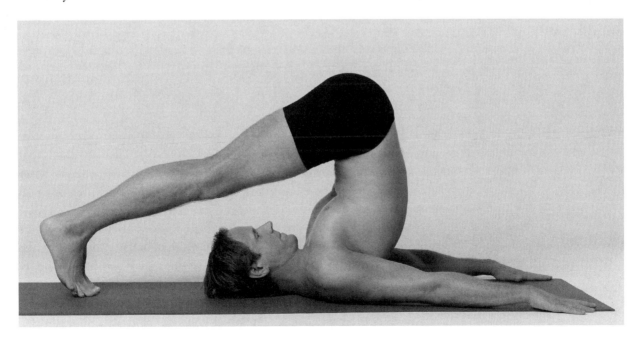

Key Actions

- Do not forget to breathe.
- Maintain an upward gaze. Remember, your neck should be elongated to be sure there is no pressure on it. Make sure you do not turn your head from side to side; it can be very harmful to your neck. If your neck feels wrong, the pose is wrong. If you feel any strain, put a blanket beneath your shoulders.

Modifications

- Beginner: You can start this pose from a prone position, if Shoulderstand does not work for you. Start at step 4 by bending at the hip joints. Plow Pose is considered an intermediate to advanced pose. If you feel strain on your neck, unroll your spine a bit and allow your hips to move down toward the front of the mat, or move your hands to your lower back. If you feel pressure in your cervical spine (neck), bend your knees and rest them on your forehead to come out of the pose. You can also do Plow Pose with your legs resting on a chair instead of touching your feet to the floor behind you.
- Intermediate: For an abdominal workout, raise your legs so they are parallel to the floor. Hold for about 5 to 10 breaths. Lower your legs back to the ground. Repeat.

Benefits

This relaxing and rejuvenating pose releases tension in your neck and shoulders. It also helps relieve insomnia and headaches by stimulating the stress-regulating thyroid gland.

Contraindications

Do not do this pose if you have neck issues, asthma, or high blood pressure, or if you are pregnant or menstruating.

Inspiration

Plow Pose only appears a bit awkward. It is actually a restful, restorative pose. Like a plow being drawn by a horse, think of your body alignment being gently drawn into place by gravity. In the process, imagine your inner core is being squeezed, just as a plow turns the earth, releasing all tension.

  If you need support, use it. Start with the highest level of support and explore your comfort level from there (note the choice of arm and hand positions offered in this pose). When doing inversions, you want to defy gravity, not common sense. This is a kernel of wisdom that should be applied to all poses at all levels.

  Always protect your neck. The older you get, the more important this becomes. Yogis are often compared to contortionists and rubber bands, but humans are not made of rubber. We are not here to stretch our ligaments. We aim to stretch our muscles, so we must be gentle and respect any physical limitations.

FEATHERED PEACOCK POSE (PINCHA MAYURASANA)

Getting In

- Start in Downward-Facing Dog Pose (Adho Mukha Svansana), with your palms flat on the floor and your hands shoulder-width apart. Keep your spine straight.
- Shifting your weight forward onto your arms, lower your forearms until they are flat on the floor with palms down and fingertips forward. Keep your elbows directly under your shoulders. Do not let your elbows splay out to the sides.
- Walk your feet in slightly.
- Step one foot forward, bend the knee, and kick the opposite leg straight up. Use strength and control to lift the second leg. Your body rises, perpendicular to the ground.
- Be careful not to sag into your shoulders.
- Hug your inner thighs together and keep your core active to maintain a sense of lightness.
- To deepen the stretch, press your forearms into the floor. Lift your abdominals in toward your spine, and lift your sit bones and tailbone. Lengthen the stretch up through your torso, legs and toes.
- Direct your gaze downward.
- Breathe deeply. Hold for several breaths or longer.
- To release, slowly and with control let one foot and then the other come back to the floor. Return to Downward-Facing Dog Pose or recline in Child's Pose (Balasana).

Key Actions

- Use your abdominals like a brace, helping you to maintain strength and balance in the pose.
- Remember those strong arms. Activate your hands, wrists, and forearms.

Modifications

- Beginner: Start by practicing Feathered Peacock Pose against a wall. Start in Downward-Facing Dog Pose, with your fingertips about 6 inches from the wall. Follow the steps already given to lift your legs. Once your legs are vertical and your body is parallel to the wall, bend your knees and place the soles of both feet against the wall. You can also keep your legs straight and rest your heels against the wall. If and when you are ready, activate your core and legs to lift your body away from the wall.

• Beginner: Conversely, build up to the pose by starting in Downward-Facing Dog Pose with your heels pressing against the wall behind you. Place your forearms flat on the floor and walk your legs up the wall until they are parallel to the ground. Walk your legs higher as you build

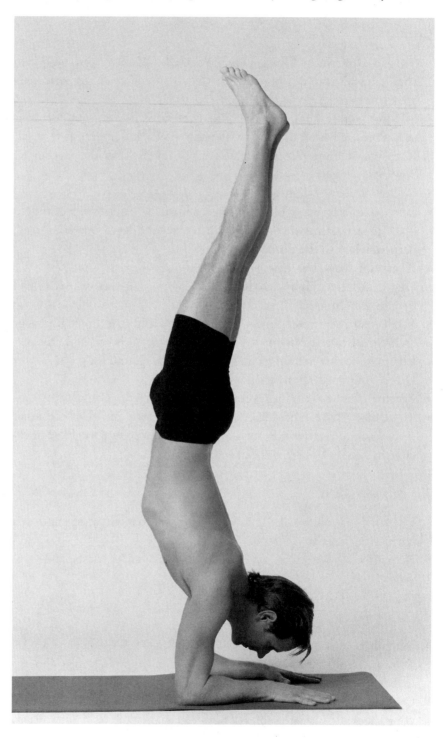

your balance and strength. Eventually try lifting one leg and then the other away from the wall.

- Intermediate: Bend your knees, arch your back, and lower your pointed toes toward the front of your head. Work toward lightly touching the soles of your feet to the crown of your head.
- Advanced: Do horizontal or vertical splits with your legs.

Benefits

A few minutes in this pose strengthens your shoulders, arms, and wrists.

Contraindications

Do not do this pose if you have high blood pressure or heart issues, or if you are pregnant or menstruating.

Inspiration

It sometimes feels natural to allow your back to curve slightly during this pose. Initially, focus on creating one straight plane perpendicular to the floor. Then go with the flow. An arch allows you to open your chest and lengthen your spine. It may be the precursor to a feet-to-head bend. But keep your core strong and never lose your center. Your spine is balanced with your center of gravity. Use your abdominal muscles as support for the bend.

SHOULDERSTAND (SALAMBA SARVANGASANA)

Getting In

- Lie on your back with your knees bent and feet on the mat.
- Drawing in your abdominal muscles, lift your legs straight up to a 90-degree angle.
- Extend your arms alongside your body with the palms down.
- Pressing down with your hands for leverage, draw your abdominals in to lift your buttocks off the floor.
- Roll your spine, vertebra by vertebra, off the mat, from your hips to your shoulders. Keep your weight on your shoulders, not your head! Align your hips with your shoulders.
- Bend your elbows and place your hands on your back for support. Brace your upper arms on the floor. To deepen the stretch, move your elbows closer together and your hands lower on your back to lengthen and lift your torso.
- Draw your abdominals in while lifting your tailbone and sit bones to lengthen the stretch. Activate your core and legs.
- Relax your neck, throat, and tongue.
- Direct your gaze upward.

- Breathe deeply. Hold for 3 breaths or longer.
- To come out, roll your spine back down to the floor.

Key Actions

- Engage your hip flexors and activate your psoas muscles. Keep your legs fully alive and activated, as this can help bring your spine to vertical.

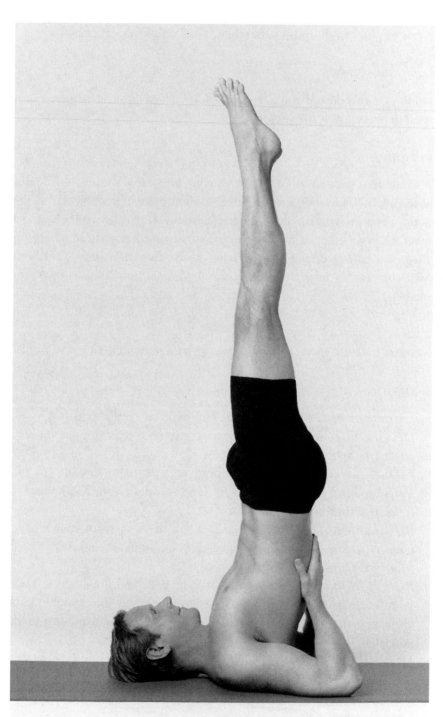

- Keep your hips stacked over your shoulders without allowing your elbows to splay out to the sides. Feel a wonderful sense of lift here.
- To protect your neck, refrain from moving your head from side to side.

Modifications

- Beginner: If you are having problems getting into the inversion, use the wall:

  Place your buttocks close to the wall and lie on your back with your legs straight up the wall, creating a 90-degree angle between your legs and torso.

  Bend your knees and place the soles of your feet flat against the wall so your shins are parallel to the ground. Begin to roll your spine off the floor, lifting your hips up above your head. Walk your feet higher up the wall.

  Gently shuffle your shoulders closer to the wall until your hips are directly over your shoulders. Place your hands on your lower back for support.

  Lift one leg straight up, directly over the hip. Alternate legs. Bring the first leg back down and lift the other one. When you are ready, lift both legs directly over your hips. Use the feet-to-wall support to help prevent your spine from collapsing.
- Beginner: If you feel comfortable away from the wall, rolling into Shoulderstand from an easy seated position provides a nice spring into the pose.
- Intermediate: Try a modified Plow Pose (Halasana). Start in Shoulderstand, then lower one leg over your head until it is parallel to the ground. Return to Shoulderstand, and lower the other leg. Continue, alternating legs, for another great abdominal workout.

Benefits

This relaxing and restorative pose rejuvenates your nervous system. It also relieves tension in your neck muscles and activates your abdominals.

Contraindications

Do not do this pose if you have neck issues or high blood pressure, or if you are pregnant or menstruating.

Inspiration

A new vantage point encourages us to think differently and expand our minds. This is a great time to be creative. Meditating while upside down can ultimately guide us to explore new perspectives that we may not have considered before. When you return to your thoughts, consider a persistent challenge that has been weighing on you, and see if you think about it any differently.

HEADSTAND (SIRSASANA)

Getting In

You can fold up your mat or pad it with a blanket to provide a more cushioned support.

- Start in Table Pose (on your hands and knees). Rest your forearms on the floor, shoulder-width apart, with your palms down.
- Interlock your fingers, keeping the thumbs up, and create a V shape with your forearms on the floor in front of you.
- Lower the top of your head to the mat, cupping the back of your head with your interlocked hands (see the Modifications section that follows).
- Press your elbows and forearms into the floor while gently stretching your neck. Relax your neck, throat, and tongue.
- Tuck your toes, lift your sit bones into the air, and walk your legs close to your torso.
- Lift one leg off the ground and bend this knee toward the sky. Let your other leg follow.
- Continue to lift your bent knees until they are directly over your hips. The soles of your feet are now facing the floor, with your heels toward your buttocks.
- Pressing your elbows and forearms into the ground, gradually straighten your legs until they are directly over your hips, with the soles of your feet facing the sky.
- Press your elbows and forearms down and draw your shoulder blades in while activating your core. Lift your tailbone and sit bones to lengthen the stretch while pressing your heels up.
- Direct your gaze straight ahead.
- Breathe deeply. Hold for 5 to 10 breaths or longer.
- To release, reverse out of the pose. To relax, come into Child's Pose (Balasana).

Key Actions

- More advanced students may choose to lift both legs at the same time, or scissor-kick one leg up and then the other. This is not a good approach for beginners. Underdevelopment of shoulder and core strength can place excessive body weight on your head, potentially causing compression in your neck.
- Rather than kicking your legs in the air, see if you can enlist your core strength. Just as in other inversions, your core performs the essential function of holding your upper and lower extremities in harmony. Make sure your pelvis is neutral, and be careful not to overarch your lower back. Engage Uddiyana Bandha (Abdominal Lock) to stabilize your pelvis and enliven your legs.

- Think of being in a standing pose: you would not let your legs just hang out. Imagine your legs and arms are in a strong Warrior Pose (Virabhadrasana), with everything energized and very much alive.
- I often see people rolling too far forward or too far back on their heads, which is unsafe for the neck and jaw. Find stability and support in your foundation—your head, elbows, forearms, and the parts of your hands that touch the floor.

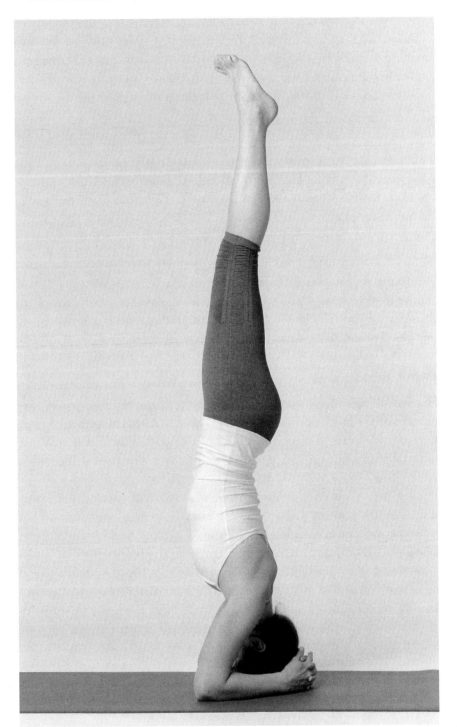

Modifications

- Beginner: If you are just beginning to practice this pose, press the bases of your palms together and snuggle the back of your head against your interlocked hands. More experienced students can open their hands and place the back of their head into their open palms. There is a temptation to kick up into this pose, like in Handstand (Adho Mukha Vrksasana) or Feathered Peacock Pose (Pincha Mayurasana), but I believe you have to earn your Headstand by coming into the pose more slowly, with greater control and precision. Unlike other inversions, where I encourage beginners to start with a wall practice, learning Headstand against a wall can be a hard habit to break. It is sometimes better to take your time and learn it without the wall.

Benefits

This pose is a head-to-toe energizer. It strengthens your arms, legs, spine, and lungs. The blood flow stimulates your brain, heart, and circulation. It also works your core, improves digestion, and tones your abdominal organs.

Contraindications

Headstand makes you vulnerable to great cervical compression. If you choose to practice it, you should have some supervision at first to ensure the safety of your alignment. It is also contraindicated if you have high or low blood pressure, or if you are pregnant or menstruating.

Inspiration

Headstand intimidates some people. If you focus on the final pose at the expense of finding the proper alignment, you can leave yourself vulnerable to injury. Take small steps and keep practicing. Gently and slowly ease into the pose while exploring your comfort zone. The pose will come to you in time.

Each person's head is different, so be very aware of your neck and how it feels in this posture. Keep your chin away from your chest, but do not jut it out too much. Imagine how you hold your chin in Mountain Pose (Tadasana). This is the same position you want in Headstand.

Some people try to find the placement of their head by measuring a certain distance from the front hairline, but my hairline changes. I cannot keep up with it! Here's a measurement trick: place the heel of your palm just above your eyebrows and place your middle finger straight up your head to find your crown.

CHAPTER 14

Backbends

BACKBENDS HELP INCREASE energy and bring confidence and courage to our lives. In bending backward, we open the front of the body, including the abdomen, hips, legs, and chest. When we stretch the abdomen, we stimulate the digestive and reproductive organs as well as the kidneys. The opening of the chest also automatically opens the lungs and the area around the heart. When we are in tune with this, we can become much more available to pure breath and to real love in our lives. The courage that lives behind our heart moves into the hearts of others in our lives.

COBRA POSE (BHUJANGASANA)

Getting In

- Lie facedown with your feet hip-width apart and the soles facing the sky.
- Place your palms under your shoulders with your fingers spread and pointing forward. Position your upper arms parallel to the floor, and hug your elbows in toward your rib cage.
- Place your forehead on the mat.
- Activate and lengthen your core, drawing your sit bones down and stretching through your thighs and calves all the way down through your toes.
- Draw your tailbone in and press your pubic bone to the mat.
- Inhale. Drawing on the strength of your abdominal muscles and thighs, lift your upper torso and head as high as you can while keeping your hips on the mat. Press your hands into the floor to heighten the lift.

- Open your chest by gently curving your spine and straightening your arms.
- Direct your gaze forward or up at the sky, whichever is comfortable for your neck.
- Hold for 5 to 10 breaths or longer.
- Maintain the alignment between your spine, neck, and head.
- Exhale and release the pose.

Key Actions

- Imagine that you are a snake. Begin the pose without using your hands to get an idea of what it feels like to slide your belly across the ground. Think of your legs as the snake's tail, and get a sense of the length that propels your body forward.
- Remember that your head only goes back as a consequence of the back-bend. It is not an initiating force, so don't just throw your head back carelessly. Be kind to your neck.
- Keep your elbows and shoulders drawn in. Do not let your arms splay to the sides.

Modifications

- Beginner: Keep your elbows bent and your upper arms in line with your upper torso. Engage your abdominal muscles and lift your torso

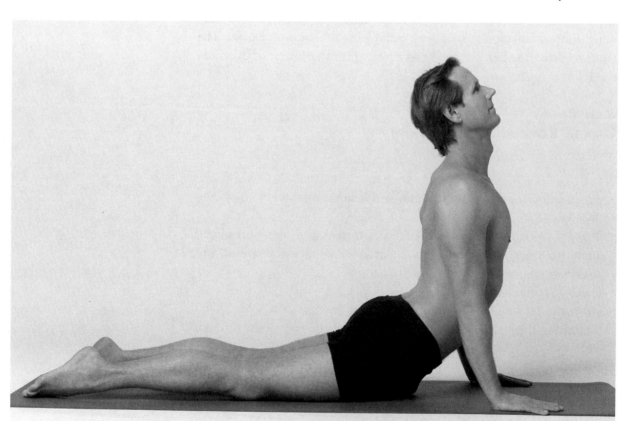

and hips off the floor. Squeeze your shoulder blades toward each other, keeping your shoulders down, and open your heart.

- Intermediate: Press your hands down, straighten your arms, and lift your chest and the fronts of your hips, allowing your torso to bend backward. Let your head fall back as you deepen the arch in your back. Keep your shoulders down away from your ears. Bend your legs up from the knees, toes pointed, and touch the soles of your feet to the crown of your head. Hold for 5 to 10 breaths or longer while breathing deeply.

Benefits

Even a small lift off the floor can give you a good stretch through your chest, lungs, abdomen, and spine. This pose also stimulates your digestive system.

Contraindications

Do not do this pose if you have back or wrist issues.

Inspiration

Students often have a misdirected preoccupation with creating an instant backbend. But without the lift, you are missing the real essence of the pose and the chance to feel the strength of your legs, spinal muscles, and core lifting you taller as you enter the pose. If you pop straight into the backbend, you miss the elegant experience of the lift. Focus on the lift first, then allow the backbend to deepen gracefully.

Bow Pose (Dhanurasana)

Getting In

- Lie facedown with your arms at your sides, palms up and fingertips pointing toward your toes. Place your chin on the mat.
- Strengthen your spine by activating the area around your navel and drawing your abdominals up and in toward your spine. Tuck your tailbone, and your weight will shift subtly onto your pelvis.
- Bend your knees, bringing your heels toward your head. Reach back with your arms and wrap your hands around your outer ankles or feet.
- Gently press your shins and feet back, away from you, as you arch into a bow shape with your whole body. As your arms and legs reach back, simultaneously lift your head, neck, and chest. Elongate your neck and tuck your chin slightly.
- Balance your weight on your abdominals. Keep your legs hip-width apart by drawing your inner thighs toward each other.

- Direct your gaze forward or up, always keeping your forehead relaxed.
- Breathe deeply. Hold for 5 to 10 breaths or longer.
- To come out, slowly lower your upper body to the floor and release your legs.

Key Actions

- There may be a tendency to let the body slump and the head and neck jam backward. It is important not to let this happen, otherwise there may be compression in the cervical spine. Make sure your knees are no wider than your hips by squeezing your inner thighs together gently. Kick your shins back as your feet lift up, using the strength of your legs, core, and arms.
- Draw your navel center in and up, as if you could lift your belly off the floor. Keep the strength in your legs.

Modifications

- Beginner: Lie on your belly and take hold of your ankles without lifting up. Finding the initial flexibility for this pose may be a challenge, especially for those who sit hunched at a desk all day. You can also start by placing your left forearm in front of your chest and parallel to the front of the mat. Place your right arm along the side of your body. Bend your right knee. Take hold of your right foot with your right hand and bend your right knee, gently drawing your heel toward your hip to stretch out the quadricep. Release, and repeat on the left side. Next, assume the bow position on one side at a time, further

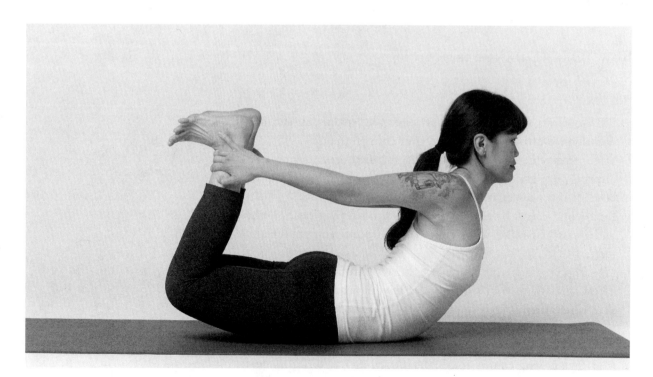

deepening the stretch. Be aware of your knees here, and try to keep them from splaying out to the sides.

Benefits

This is a good stretch for the front of your body, and it provides a nice flex for your spine. It also strengthens your back, quads, and abdominal muscles.

Contraindications

Do not do this pose if you have high or low blood pressure or neck or lower back issues.

Inspiration

A common question is whether or not to "squeeze your butt" in Bow Pose. A simple answer: if you are squeezing and it hurts your back, stop! But if it is comfortable, give it a try. Yoga is about creating a state of *ahimsa*, the practice of doing less harm in our lives. If we are too gung ho about trying to get each pose perfect, our overambition will be counterproductive and may end up doing more harm than good.

ONE-LEGGED KING PIGEON POSE (EKA PADA RAJAKAPOTASANA)

Getting In

- Start in Downward-Facing Dog Pose (Adho Mukha Svansana).
- Bend your right knee and bring it forward, placing it slightly to the right of your right wrist so the shin is as close to parallel to the front edge of the mat as possible.
- Check your alignment: your right knee should be in front of your right hip. Flex your right toes toward your shin.
- Simultaneously extend your left leg back until the knee is resting on the mat.
- Position your hands beside or in front of your hips. Center your spine over the tripod created by your tailbone and sit bones.
- Fold your torso forward and walk your hands out in front. Either rest your forearms on the floor with your hands in prayer position, or extend your arms completely and rest your forehead on the mat.
- Feel the stretch in your groins. Deepen the stretch by lowering your hips closer to the floor.
- Direct your gaze forward.
- Breathe deeply. Hold for 5 to 10 breaths or longer.
- Release back into Downward-Facing Dog Pose, and repeat on the other side.

Key Actions

- A lot of the action begins with your back foot. Gently press the lateral (outside) part of your foot down. This can really help level your hips and allows your back thigh to roll in.
- Square off your hips to take any potential strain off your lower back. If you are having a hard time squaring your hips, straighten your spine and raise up on your hands or fingertips to lift out of your pelvis.
- Keep your hips moving downward and feel a lifting sensation from your lower back. (This is where core engagement helps.)
- This one-legged balancing act can be a resting pose. If you are enjoying the forward fold and hip opening, stay folded down. Relax and surrender to the pose.

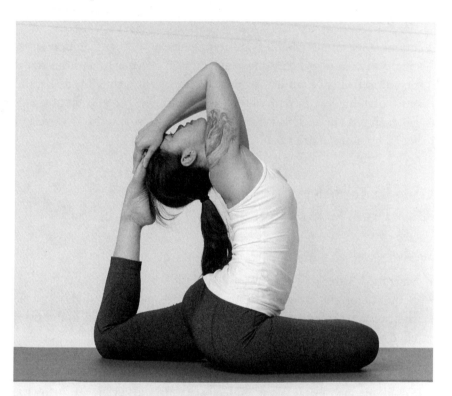

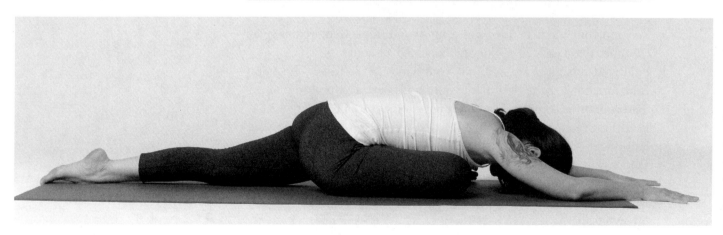

Modifications

- Beginner: If this pose causes pain in your bent front knee, a good modification is Thread the Needle Pose (Parsva Balasana). Roll onto your back and hug your right knee into your chest. Place your left foot on the floor with your knee bent. Cross your right ankle over your left thigh, and gently guide your right knee open. If this feels okay, you can hug your left knee into your chest while continuing to flex your right foot. If there is still no discomfort, take your right arm through the space between your legs and your left arm outside your left leg to clasp hands, either behind your left thigh or on top of your left shin. Gently draw your legs in closer to your torso while moving your right thigh away. Hold for 5 to 10 breaths or longer. Repeat on the other side.
- Intermediate: From One-Legged King Pigeon Pose, bend your back knee at a right angle until your toe is pointed toward the sky. Raise both arms straight above you with your palms facing back. Bend your elbows until your hands can take hold of your foot.
- Advanced: Draw your foot toward your head.

Benefits

This is a super stretch for your thighs, groins, and psoas muscles. It also opens your shoulders and chest.

Contraindications

Do not do this pose if you have high or low blood pressure or ankle or knee issues.

Inspiration

It is great to be graceful and poetic in this pose, but be careful not to get fixated on what it looks like from the outside. As you deepen the stretch, focus on the deeper meaning behind the pose and your practice. Try not to abandon the basic guidelines of *ahimsa*. There are so many things going on in this pose, and you are asking your body to do a lot from every angle. It is fundamental to be fully aware of all this activity instead of focusing on just one part of it. Yogic breathing helps center the activity and energize your whole body. The grace and ease of this pose comes through with your breath and your intention.

FISH POSE (MATSYASANA)

Getting In

- Lie on your back with your arms down by your sides. Slide your hands under your buttocks, palms down. Extend your legs and flex your feet.

- Draw your shoulder blades down your back and begin to open your chest before lifting your torso off the mat.
- Drawing your abdominal muscles in, lift your torso and head to look at your toes. Bend your elbows, placing your weight on your forearms while simultaneously bringing your upper arms perpendicular to the floor. Keep your hands firmly tucked under your buttocks.
- Gently drop your head back, lowering the crown of your head to the mat. Keep your weight primarily on your elbows and forearms, *not* on your head. Draw in your abdominal muscles to keep the weight on your head to a minimum.
- Squeeze your upper thighs together. Extend out through the balls of your feet. Press your palms and forearms into the floor to deepen the arch and open your chest.
- Extend your chin back slightly to elongate your neck. Relax your neck and throat.
- Direct your gaze up or behind you.
- Breathe deeply. Hold for 5 to 10 breaths or longer.
- To release, make sure your core is engaged, lift your head toward your toes, and slowly lower your torso to the mat.

Key Actions

- Once in the pose, roll your shoulders up and then down.
- To avoid sagging into your shoulders, place equal attention on your elbows and palms. Press your elbows, forearms, and palms down to eliminate any collapse in your shoulders and aid in opening your chest.
- It is fun to explore opening your throat and taking a liberating Ujjayi breath here.

Modifications

- Beginner: Bend your knees and place your feet flat on the floor, hip-width apart. To focus your weight, press your palms into the

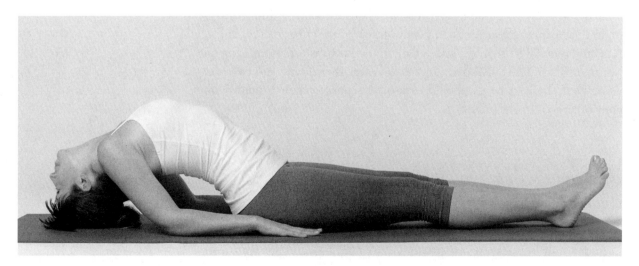

ground and strengthen your arms. Avoid placing too much weight on your head.

Benefits

This is both a relaxing and an invigorating stretch through your abdominals, chest, and back. It also improves your posture and opens your throat.

Contraindications

Do not do this pose if you have a migraine, insomnia, high blood pressure, or neck issues. If you have low blood pressure, keep your chin tucked as you lift your chest; do not collapse your head back.

Inspiration

The safest guide to protecting your neck is maintaining awareness. Notice when a position is comfortable or uncomfortable. Find a place where you feel supported in the pose. Distribute approximately 25 percent of your weight to your neck. But if it hurts, back off.

LOCUST POSE (SALABHASANA)

Getting In

- Lie facedown with your arms by your sides, palms up and fingertips pointing toward your toes. Keep the tops of your feet on the mat with toes pointed, and bring your legs and ankles together.
- Rest your forehead on the mat. Relax your body for a moment, surrendering to the earth.
- Tuck your tailbone and press your pelvis down. Exhale completely.
- Inhale. Simultaneously lift your legs, arms, and chest off the ground. Elongate your arms with your fingers pointing toward your toes. Lift your torso and straight legs into a bow.
- Direct your gaze forward by slightly lifting your chin, but do not overextend the neck. If you feel tension in your neck, gaze down and draw your chin slightly toward your chest.
- Stretch your fingertips back toward your toes. Draw your shoulder blades in and down your back as you open your chest.
- With your weight on your abdominals and pelvis, engage your core by drawing your abdominals up and in to lengthen and heighten the pose.
- Breathe deeply. Hold for several breaths or longer.
- To release, lower your torso and limbs to the ground. Rest your arms on the mat alongside you and turn your head to one side. Touch your big toes together.

Key Actions

- Tap into your leg strength here. Some instructors advise keeping your legs apart, but I like keeping them long and together. This creates a strong single "tail" that is a lot easier to lift. Consider an internal rotation of your thighs, where the inner thighs rotate toward the sky.
- Your head and neck must be comfortable; you can look down and slightly in front of you, look at the sky, or look straight ahead.

Modifications

- Beginner: If you are straining to lift both legs, lift one leg at a time. Lower it, and repeat on the other side. If you are straining your lower back, place your hands on the floor under your shoulders—similar to Cobra Pose (Bhujangasana)—and lift your legs and torso.
- Intermediate: Change your arm position by interlocking your fingers behind your back or extending your arms out in front of you like Superman. (In fact, this pose is called Superhero Pose.)
- Advanced: Deepen the bow position by reaching back with both arms, taking hold of your ankles, and moving into Bow Pose (Dhanurasana).

Benefits

This is a workout for both mind and body. It stretches your shoulders, back, and thighs while energizing your mind.

Contraindications

Do not do this pose if you have a headache or back issues.

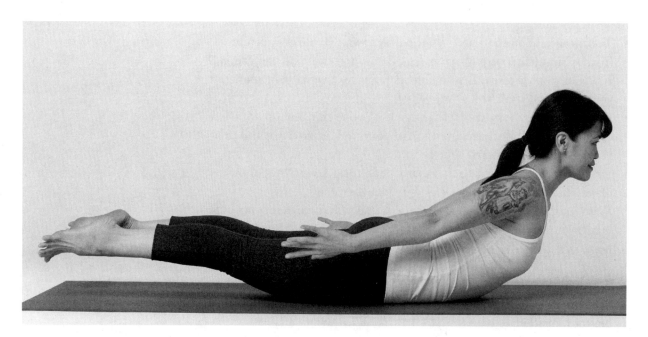

Inspiration

The challenge here is to stay present and not obsess over the end result or want the pose to be over. Give yourself the benefit of exploring the lengthening of your legs. If you find yourself mentally fading or panicking, change something. Whether it is your body, your breath, or just your mind, it will make a difference.

Bridge Pose (Setu Bandha Sarvangasana)

Getting In

- Lie on your back with your knees bent; your feet flat on the floor about hip-width apart; and your arms by your sides, palms down. The outer edges of your feet should be parallel to the outer edges of your mat.
- Align your heels with your sit bones. Touch the backs of your heels with your fingertips.
- Inhale as you press your feet into the floor and lift your pubic bone and tailbone as high as is comfortable. Keep your knees hip-width apart.
- Lift your chest toward your chin while lifting your chin slightly away from your chest to maintain the natural curve in your neck.
- Lengthen the stretch through your neck, spine, and thighs.
- Press your feet evenly into the ground.
- Deepen the stretch by clasping your hands underneath you, drawing your shoulder blades together, and extending your arms toward your heels.
- Direct your gaze up toward the sky.
- Breathe deeply. Hold for 5 to 10 breaths or longer.

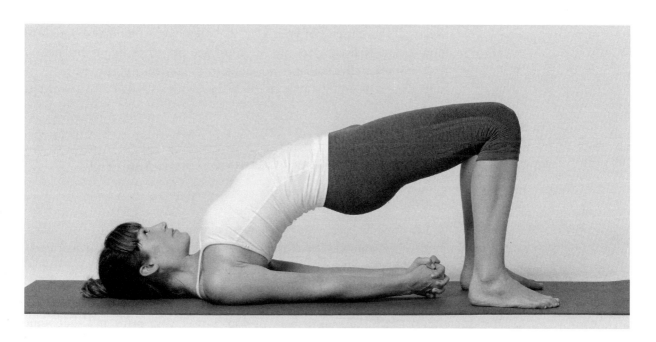

- To release, exhale and lower your torso vertebra by vertebra, moving down from upper to middle to lower spine.

Key Actions

- The action of the muscles changes as you transition from moving into the pose to actually being in it. When you lift up into the pose, engage your glutes. However, once you are in the pose, let your legs and core take over. This movement requires quite a bit of focus, but it *is* doable.
- Do not completely relax your buttocks. Keep your glutes working, but not so much that you create compression in your lower back.

Modifications

- Beginner: Rest your sacrum on a bolster for support.
- Intermediate: Place your hands under your hips with your weight on your upper arms. Extend one leg straight up and point and flex the toes. Bring it down and switch legs. Hold for 5 breaths for each leg.

Benefits

This pose provides a comfortable stretch through your chest, neck, hips, and spine. It also helps with digestion, fatigue, and stress and stimulates your thyroid.

Contraindications

Do not do this pose if you have lower back or neck issues.

Inspiration

Relax all the muscles of your face, and allow your blood and breath to flow freely. Releasing tension in your face improves blood circulation and skin elasticity. If that is not enough to convince you to relax, consider this: tension in your face can add as many as ten years to your appearance!

UPWARD BOW POSE (URDHVA DHANURASANA)

Getting In

- Lie on your back with your knees bent and arms down by your sides. Position your feet flat on the floor about hip-width apart and your heels against your sit bones. The outer edges of your feet should be parallel to the outer edges of your mat.
- Lift your arms toward the sky and bend your elbows so your forearms face the wall in back of you. Lower your arms and slide your

hands under your shoulders with your palms on the ground and fingers splayed. Hug your elbows in toward each other.

- Inhale. Press your feet into the floor and lift your pubic bone and tailbone as high as is comfortable.
- Press into your hands and rise up onto the crown of your head. Straighten your arms and legs, lifting your head off the ground as you rise farther into a bow shape. Elongate your neck, feeling the stretch through the crown of your head as it reaches toward the ground.
- Keep your toes from turning out by pressing evenly through your feet.
- Direct your gaze toward the back wall or down toward the mat between your hands.
- Hold for several breaths.
- Exhale and lower to the back of your head and then to your torso, moving from upper to middle to lower spine, back to the mat.

Key Actions

- Turn your upper arms outward but keep your weight on the base of your index fingers and inner thumbs.
- If you are already limber and open in the shoulders, back off your shoulders and focus more on strength in your legs.

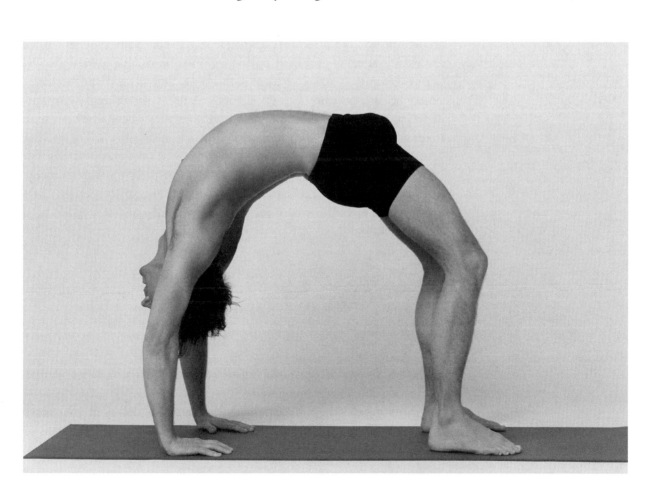

- Feel your feet and the opening in your groins.

- Lift your hips toward the sky as you draw more strength into your legs.

Modifications

- Intermediate: Practice bending your elbows to lower the crown of your head toward the floor, rising back up, and then lowering again. If this hurts your neck, keep your head slightly off the mat.
- Advanced: If Upward Bow Pose feels easy, walk your feet closer to your head.

Benefits

This pose helps lengthen and realign your back as it stretches your chest, spine, and lungs. It also strengthens your arms, wrists, and legs.

Contraindications

Do not do this pose if you have wrist or lower back issues or high blood pressure.

Inspiration

Many students doubt their ability to come into this pose. Have faith! The average person *can* do a full backbend. If you take your time and work toward it gradually, your belly button will soon be arching toward the sky. Start by simply picturing yourself in this pose. Often, we are unsuccessful simply because we cannot imagine ourselves doing something. Many students have the individual components, but then they freeze when it is time to lift up. You may feel disoriented as you move upside down. Try walking your hands under your shoulders, and then visualize yourself lifting up. Next, use the strength of your arms and legs to press up incrementally. After two or three attempts, you may be amazed to finally experience lift-off. You have already pictured the pose, so you can do it. Yoga begins with the imagination.

UPWARD-FACING DOG POSE (URDHVA MUKHA SVANASANA)

Getting In

- Lie facedown with your legs hip-width apart, the tops of your feet on the mat, and your toes pointed.
- Bend your elbows and place your hands, palms down, at your sides under your shoulders. Splay your fingers. Avoid relaxing your arms to the side; instead, draw your elbows in toward your rib cage.

- Inhale. Straighten your arms and lift your body off the mat. Lift your knees and thighs as well. Put your weight on your hands and the tops of your feet.
- Roll your hips forward, drawing in your abdominals and strengthening your thighs. Let your thighs rotate inward slightly.
- Lengthen the stretch and take the pressure off your lower back by tucking your tailbone down toward the floor, elongating your spine, pressing your shoulders back and down, and opening your chest. Lengthen your neck away from your shoulders.
- Direct your gaze forward or up toward the sky.
- Breathe deeply. Hold for 5 to 10 breaths or longer.
- To release, bend your knees and place them on the mat. Bend your elbows and slowly, with control, lower onto your stomach.

Key Actions

- This pose is less about the actual backbend than it is about the lifting action that creates the backbend. If you compromise the lift, you miss the essential foundation of the pose.
- Press your hands into the floor and let your shoulders roll back and down, allowing a sensation of lightness and strength to permeate the pose.
- To avoid lower back stress, keep your hands aligned under your shoulders and your core engaged.

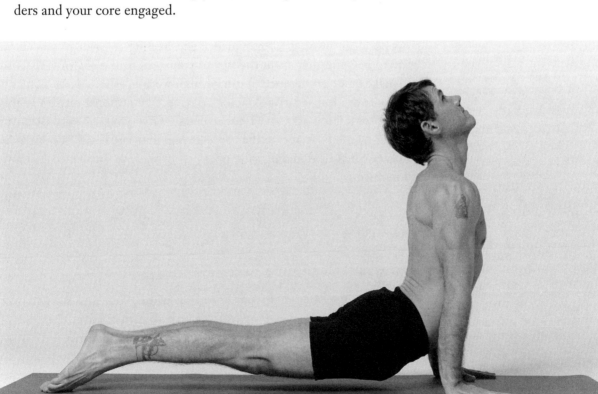

- Don't hunch your shoulders up to your ears. Instead, press your hands into the floor, allowing your arms to be straight and strong.
- Relax your face and jaw in this pose. Remember to bring joy and lightness to it, and avoid tensing or gripping.

Modifications

- Beginner: Build strength in Cobra Pose (Bhujangasana) and eventually move on to Upward-Facing Dog Pose. Gradually work toward lifting your thighs and knees, fully elevating your body until only your hands and the tops of your feet are on the ground.
- Intermediate: Start from the top of a push-up, lower yourself by bending your elbows alongside your rib cage, and move from there into Upward-Facing Dog Pose. Hold for 5 to 10 breaths or longer.

Benefits

This pose presents a good opportunity to tone your core. It strengthens your back, stretches your chest, and stimulates your abdominal organs.

Contraindications

Do not do this pose if you have lower back or wrist issues.

Inspiration

This pose can bring great confidence and healing. Allowing your entire body to become alive from the tips of your toes to the top of your head will make quite a difference. It can be empowering, especially in moments when you are lost, heartbroken, or grieving. My personal mantra in this pose is something akin to "I am soaring." Give yourself permission to let your whole body feel unified as a strong, buoyant vessel of pure love, with your heart lifted and wide open, allowing love and grace to move through you.

CAMEL POSE (USTRASANA)

Getting In

- Kneel on your mat with your knees hip-width, your hips stacked over your knees, and your shoulders stacked over your hips. The tops of your feet should be on the mat with your toes pointed back.
- Prepare for the backbend by activating your thighs. Point your chin up slightly. Tuck your tailbone, lengthen your spine, and elongate your neck away from your shoulders.
- Place your hands on your lower back, drawing your elbows back to open your chest.

- To protect your lower back, draw in your abdominal muscles and keep them strong.
- Reach back with your right hand, bringing the fingertips or palm to rest on your right heel. Follow with your left hand. Your hips may move slightly forward, but take care not to press them too far forward past your knees.
- Deepen the arch in your back. Leading with the crown of your head, keep your abdominals drawing in and gradually stretch your head back while maintaining your neck's alignment with your spine.
- Feel your heart center lift up as you draw the backbend more into your thoracic (mid) spine and out of your lumbar (lower) spine.
- Breathe deeply. Hold for 5 to 10 breaths or longer.
- To release, return your hands to your lower back and draw on your abdominal muscles. Lead from your chest to return to a kneeling position. Lift your head last.

Key Actions

- As you come into the backbend, the gaze moves from the wall in front of you to the one in back. The key is to make sure your neck is supported without the slightest bit of strain.
- Often, students try to go too far too quickly in this backbend, and the alignment of their hips over their knees collapses. Stack your hips over your knees and keep your quads strong. As you reach back for your

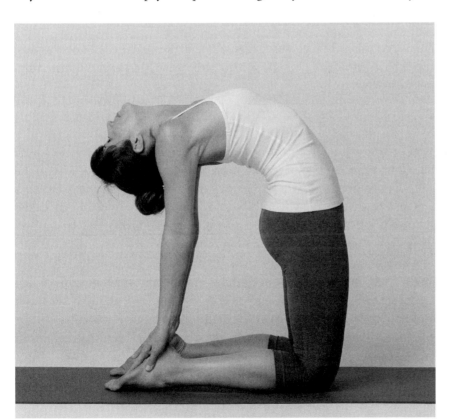

heels, use your core strength to protect your back. Activation of your core is even more important when you come out of the pose.

- Keep your thighs working and do not collapse the strong foundation.
- While keeping your thighs hip-width apart, move them energetically toward each other so they do not collapse outward.

Modifications

- Beginner: Instead of worrying about reaching back for your heels, keep your hands on your lower back and, with a tall spine, use your thumbs to massage your lower back. As a next step, tuck your toes under to bring your heels a little higher off the ground.
- Beginner: There are three stages to every pose, and they all deserve equal attention: getting into the pose, being in the pose, and getting out of the pose. Try to maintain mindfulness equally during every stage. Above all, avoid lifting hastily out of a pose. This is when the greatest amount of harm can occur.
- Beginner: If you feel any strain when you drop your head back, keep your neck where it's most comfortable for you.

Benefits

This pose opens your chest, strengthens your back, and stretches your psoas muscles.

Contraindications

Do not do this pose if you have high blood pressure or back or neck issues. If you have low blood pressure, do not drop your head back, and rise from this pose slowly.

Inspiration

Your breath will tell you if you are in good enough form to stay in a pose for a long time. Instead of forcing your way into it, find the pose with the help of your breath. It will happen organically, so proceed with enthusiasm and trust, and allow it to blossom. Feel the lift of your heart to the sky, and think of someone you love supporting and lifting you, letting you know that whatever you have to offer is enough.

As I prepare for this pose, I stand on my knees, bring my hands to my lower back, and massage the muscles around my lumbar spine. I tell my lower back that I promise to be careful and loving and that I will not do it any harm. This mantra helps me to dispel fear. If possible, use the *drishti* (gazing point) to help you look up and then back. Sometimes to move a bit ahead in this life, it's okay to look back. Let go of fear.

CHAPTER 15

Seated Poses and Twists

Seated Poses

It's important to maintain a straight spine in many of these poses. In doing so, you can safely stretch the muscles along your spine. Just remember: Happy spine, happy life.

FIRE LOG POSE/DOUBLE PIGEON POSE (AGNISTAMBHASANA)

Getting In

- Start in Staff Pose (Dandasana; page 196), sitting on the floor with your legs straight out in front of you.
- Bend your left leg and let it fall gently out to the side, sliding your left calf under your right knee so that your left shin is parallel to the front edge of the mat.
- Place your right shin on top of your left, with your knees and ankles stacked.
- Slide both ankles just to the outside of your knees, so your right (top) anklebone is just outside your left (bottom) knee and vice versa.
- Flex both feet and tilt your pelvis forward.
- Your shins should look like stacked fire logs, with the space between the insides of your legs forming a triangle.
- Press your hands down alongside your hips while lengthening your spine, and feel your spine growing tall and centered on your sit bones.
- Keep your right anklebone outside your left thigh. This is safer for your knee and facilitates a deeper hip opening.
- Keep your feet flexed, with your heels pressing away from each other.

- Keep your core engaged, your chest lifted, your spine straight, and your shoulders away from your ears.
- Direct your gaze forward.
- Breathe deeply. Hold for 5 to 10 breaths or longer.
- Reverse legs and repeat.

Key Actions

- Instead of forcing the knee of your upper leg down, continue to build more stability in your bottom leg.
- Stay a bit longer on the side where you experience more tightness.

Modifications

- Beginner: Place blocks or a blanket under your sit bones to raise your hips higher than your knees.
- Intermediate: Place your hands in front of your knees while moving into a forward bend from your hips instead of your waist. As you tilt forward from your hips, keep your spine straight and your chest reaching forward so that both the front and back of your torso are long. Once in the forward bend, further deepen the stretch by placing your

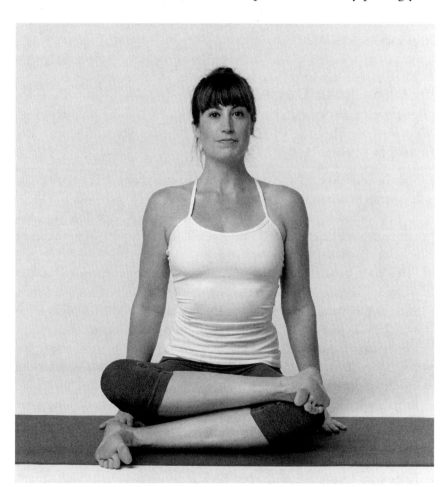

forearms on the mat in front of you. You may wish to place your palms together in prayer position.

- Intermediate: Or extend your arms behind you and clasp your hands behind your sit bones to feel a deeper hip and chest stretch.
- Intermediate: Or slide your top shin forward and away from your hip, keeping your foot flexed.

Benefits

This pose stretches your hips and groins; helps protect your knees from injury by stretching your hips, legs, and calves; and relieves tension.

Contraindications

Do not do this pose if you have lower back or knee issues.

Inspiration

In Fire Log Pose, like all poses, your mind-set is important. As its name suggests, this pose provides an opportunity to work on the solar plexus (*manipura*) chakra. The yin of this chakra is its association with fire, or stress and anger; its yang is mental health and well-being. The Fire Log Pose is known for releasing not only physical tightness but also mental tightness that manifests as tension and stress. Remember that it is our thoughts that create stress and tightness. To restore your energy flow and reduce stress, mental and physical relaxation should be performed together.

Just when you want to come out of the pose, a priceless benefit of staying in position is seeing what is on the other side of the mental process. That is where the intrigue begins and the true essence of the pose resides. Remember, people who are more flexible often have further to go, because while they are in a physically deeper expression of the pose, they may not feel it as deeply. People who are less limber are lucky! They don't have to go as far to feel the intensity of the pose.

Often, we hold on to old notions and beliefs about our own limitations, such as *I am a tight hip person*, instead of just opening to the possibilities. That's why it is great to be a beginner. You do not know what you can and cannot do.

BOUND ANGLE POSE/BUTTERFLY POSE (BADDHA KONASANA)

Getting In

- Start in Staff Pose (Dandasana; page 196), sitting on the floor with your legs straight out in front of you.
- Bend your knees, place your feet flat on the mat, and bring your heels together.

- Wrap your hands around the front of your knees and gently guide your legs closer to your body.
- Place your palms or fingertips on the floor behind your sit bones, while lifting and expanding your spine and chest.
- Let your knees splay simultaneously to the sides as the soles of your feet come together. Take hold of your feet with your hands, and guide your heels closer to your pelvis.
- Use your hands to press the soles of your feet together.
- Press your sit bones into the ground as you lengthen your spine and crown of your head.
- Bow forward with a flat back.
- Direct your gaze forward.
- Breathe deeply. Hold for 5 to 10 breaths or longer.
- To release, gently lift your torso, still keeping your back flat. Straighten your spine and return to Staff Pose.

Key Actions

- There is a misconception that the objective of this pose is to get your head to touch the floor. If you lower your head before you are ready, your hips will lift slightly, and you will miss out on an optimal stretch. Instead, focus on pressing your hips back and down. Lengthen your spine and engage your core. Now your lower back becomes active, your spine extends out of your pelvis, and your legs stay strong.
- Instead of pressing your knees down, consider using your elbows to encourage more downward action from your *thighs* as your chest moves forward and out.

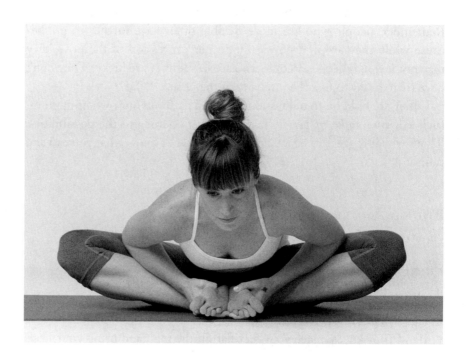

- Avoid rounding your spine. If your back begins to round, come out of the pose a little. Opening your chest and shoulders will help lift and lengthen your spine.
- If you are tight in the groin area, place a block or blanket under your sit bones for extra support.

Modifications

- Beginner: If your knees do not like this pose, engage your glutes to see if that helps relieve the discomfort. If you are feeling pain anywhere, change something immediately. If it feels wrong, it *is* wrong.
- Intermediate: If you want to make the pose more interesting, use your hands to open your feet "like a book" for a great stretch through your hips and groins.
- Advanced: Take the stretch even deeper by folding forward from your hips until your chest and head touch the mat in front of your feet. Once you are resting your forehead on the mat, extend your arms behind you, with your palms facing up and your arms resting on the floor. Or place your hands on the floor in front of you and begin to walk your hands forward while simultaneously pressing your hips back.

Benefits

This pose opens your hips, thighs, and groin and promotes prostate health. It helps to relieve the symptoms of menstruation and menopause and has often been helpful in prenatal yoga.

Contraindications

Do not do this pose if you have groin or knee issues.

Inspiration

People often use this pose as an opportunity to daydream. I believe that no pose is that simple. If you can space out, you are missing something. There is always something to do. There is always an opportunity to be fully present by connecting even more powerfully to the breath. It is often during simple poses that students, while focusing the mind, break through to new frontiers in their practice. In simplicity, there is great strength.

In yoga, it is a mistake to equate the level of difficulty with the benefits of a pose. When I see a student slacking off in Butterfly Pose, I am reminded of the butterfly effect: a small change in one place can have large effects elsewhere. Just as a butterfly flapping its wings can cause small atmospheric changes that can influence wind and weather many miles away, Butterfly Pose stimulates many organs and, in traditional texts, was believed to destroy disease.

DANDASANA (STAFF POSE)

Getting In

- Sit on the floor with your legs straight out in front of you and your feet flexed.
- Shift your weight to the front of your sit bones. Imagine using your hands to draw your buttocks back so your pelvis begins to tip forward slightly.
- Place your palms or fingertips on the mat by your sides.
- Strengthen your thighs, pressing your hamstrings into the floor without hyperextending your knees.
- Draw in your abdominals and lift out of your groins. Lift up through your whole spine while drawing your shoulder blades down your back.
- To deepen the stretch, flex your feet and press out through your heels.
- Direct your gaze forward, with your chin slightly down.
- Breathe deeply. Hold for 5 to 10 breaths or longer.

Key Actions

- Your shoulders should be aligned over your hips.
- Keep your knees pointing up while rotating your thighs slightly inward.

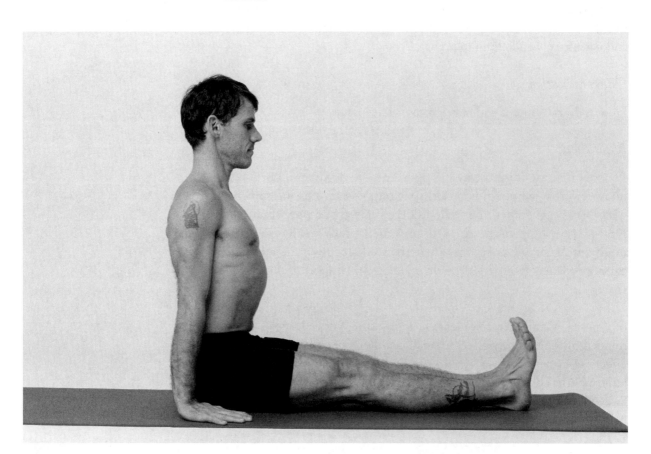

- Some folks feel their arms are too short or too long for this pose. This is a myth! Try to keep your arms straight, placing your hands beside your hips or slightly forward. You can press your palms flat on the floor or touch your fingertips if your palms won't reach.
- If you need a rest, place both hands behind you, lean back with a straight spine, and take a deep breath as you feel your chest expand. Or lean forward with a straight spine and rest your hands on your shins.

Modifications

- Intermediate: To really strengthen your legs, lift your heels off the mat. Maintain the lift, or raise (inhale) and lower (exhale) your legs with your breath. You can also engage in some foot stretches: point and hold, and then flex and hold.
- Advanced: To complete the pose, engage the *bandhas*.

Benefits

This core pose strengthens your legs and back, stretches your chest, and improves your posture, setting the foundation for other seated poses.

Contraindications

Do not do this pose if you have wrist or lower back issues.

Inspiration

This pose sets a powerful foundation for all seated poses, yet it is one of the most popular poses for fidgeting. Students underestimate its importance as they wait for something else to happen that is more dynamic or exciting. Rest in stillness and enjoy the powerful benefits of the pose. The outer discipline of strengthening your legs and core leads to inner awareness and calm.

It is, as always, important to get the form right from the beginning. Anytime you are reluctant to do a pose, ask yourself why. If you are running away from something, yoga is a great place to feel safe and check it out more closely. It could be your new best friend. Yoga often teaches us something we have not yet figured out.

COW FACE POSE (GOMUKHASANA)

Getting In

- Start in Staff Pose (Dandasana), sitting on the floor with your legs straight out in front of you and your feet flexed.
- Bend your knees.
- Slide your left foot under your right leg all the way to the outside of your right hip.

- Lift your right foot up over your left knee and place your right foot to the outside of your left hip.
- Stack your right knee on top of your left.
- Raise your left hand straight up in the air with the palm facing back.
- Bend your left elbow and slide your hand down between your shoulder blades.
- Wrap your right hand behind your back, with the palm facing away from you, and reach up your spine. If possible, interlock the fingers of your hands.
- Bend forward, lowering your upper torso toward your knees while lengthening your spine.
- Direct your gaze slightly forward and down.
- Breathe deeply. Hold for 5 to 10 breaths or longer.
- To come out, sit upright, release your arms and legs, and return to Staff Pose.
- Reverse legs and repeat the pose.

Key Actions

- Ensure that you are centered, with your weight evenly distributed on your sit bones and both feet.
- Continue to gently press back with your hips while drawing in your abdominals. Feel a nice strengthening and stretching in your lower back. Gently press your top knee into your bottom knee, building strength in your quads.
- Keep your core engaged to protect your lower back.
- Only fold forward if it feels right. In forward bends, your lower abdominals should make contact with your thigh first, then your upper abdominals and chest follow.

Modifications

- Beginner: Sometimes I think they created this arm position so we would stop thinking about our hips. It becomes a distraction. If the arm variation is too much, try bringing your hands to your hip creases, and use your fingers to facilitate Uddiyana Bandha (Abdominal Lock). Or, if you are unable to bring your hands together behind you, use a strap as a connector between your hands. It is easier to get into this position from Double Pigeon Pose, sliding both feet toward the opposite, outer hips until your knees are stacked. If the stretch in your legs and hips is too intense, place your shins parallel to the front edge of the mat instead of placing your feet beside your hips.
- Intermediate: Rest your sit bones on your feet and stack your bottom leg under the top. Or slide your feet away from your hips until both shins are parallel to the front edge of the mat, with your feet stretching as far apart as possible.

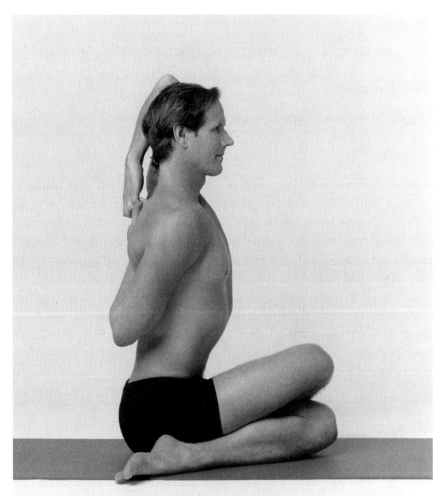

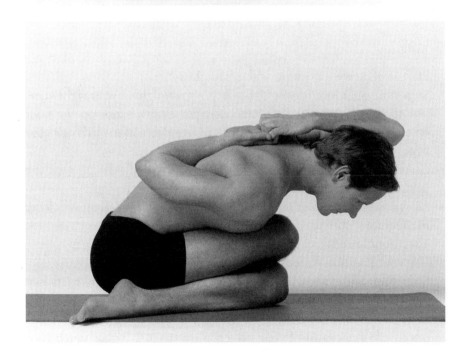

Benefits

This pose strengthens and stretches your hips, shoulders, and triceps.

Contraindications

Do not do this pose if you have knee or shoulder issues.

Inspiration

Balance can be a struggle here. If you feel unbalanced, put your hands on the floor in front of you or alongside your body. If your primary focus in the pose is trying to stay upright, make adjustments so you can breathe more deeply and rhythmically. Adjust your position so your attention is focused less on trying not to fall over and more on the strength and stillness of the pose. If you feel inclined to fall over—go for it! Gracefully, of course.

Although it seems counterintuitive, the poses with the most contortions often introduce the greatest balance and inner calmness. If you think about it, this makes perfect sense. Your arms, legs, hips, thighs, and core are engaged in this balancing act. Imagine that you look like a cow's face from above. Once balance is achieved, it is harmony.

MONKEY POSE (HANUMANASANA)

This pose is dedicated to the sage Hanuman, the monkey king. A loyal devotee to Lord Rama, Hanuman leaped across the sea from India to Sri Lanka to reassure Rama's wife, Sita, that she would be rescued from her captor, Ravana.

Getting In

- Start in a kneeling position with a straight spine.
- Step your right foot forward, then begin to straighten your right knee, sliding your hips back. Simultaneously place both hands on the floor on either side of your right foot, leaning your torso forward over your knee. This is the preliminary position for this pose.
- Continue to move your right foot and leg forward, leading with the heel, and at the same time, begin to straighten your left leg.
- As you extend your legs in opposite directions, your pelvis moves closer to the floor.
- Your right knee is facing the sky, and the left is facing the earth.
- Use your hands to control your descent.
- Straighten both legs, with your hips squared, the toes of your left foot pointed, and your right foot flexed.
- When you reach the full extension of both legs, bring your spine upright, with the crown of your head toward the sky. Either touch your hands to the floor or reach up to the sky.

- Hold for 5 to 10 breaths or longer.
- Slowly release and return to a kneeling position.
- Repeat the pose on the other side.

Key Actions

- A lot of students get hung up on the front leg and feel humbled at what they perceive as a tight hamstring. I find it interesting to let the front leg be as it is. Bring your awareness to your back leg. Start to feel your back thigh rotate inward and the back baby toe get longer and flatter on the floor. Focus on your left baby toenail, pressing it down and reaching it back. See if that takes away any resistance you may encounter in your front leg.
- Let your hamstrings guide you. If a hamstring is too tight, ease off. You can gently deepen the stretch as you breathe.
- In addition to extending your feet in opposite directions, focus on drawing the energy of your legs toward your midline, as if you could hug your thighbones into your pelvis.
- Students are often drawn to bowing forward in this pose. If you are going to take even the slightest hint of a forward fold, first lift your chest and remind yourself to keep lengthening your spine as you bow. Remember, in every forward fold, there is the essence of a backbend.

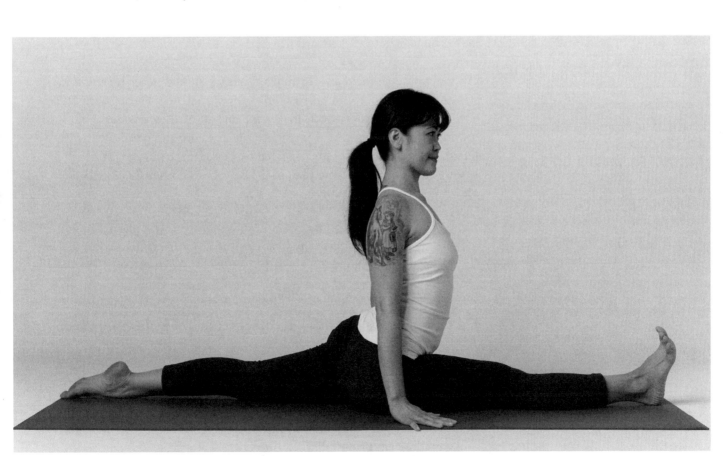

Modifications

- Beginner: If your hips are off the ground, keep your fingertips or palms down, or slide blocks under your hands for more support. Once you feel stable, especially if both your hips are close to or resting on the mat, bring your hands into prayer position at your heart. When you feel secure, reach your arms over your head. But remember: there is no rush. You can build this pose over time.
- Intermediate: To deepen the stretch, fold forward over your front leg and place your forearms on the mat.
- Advanced: Clasp your left wrist with your right hand just beyond your right foot and press your arms forward, with your right palm facing away to deepen the stretch. Alternatively, take hold of your big toe, shin, or ankle. More limber students often skip the lunge and move right into the splits position.

Benefits

This is a fun pose that stretches your thighs, hamstrings, and groins as you work on increasing flexibility.

Contraindications

Do not do this pose if you have groin or hamstring issues.

Inspiration

We may not able to fly like Hanuman, but we should never be afraid to see where our bodies can take us. Sometimes students plateau just a few centimeters from the floor. It makes me curious if they are afraid of allowing something to take place, to get deeper into the pose. Often, we limit ourselves by getting stuck in what we perceive we can and cannot do. Are we afraid of completing the pose? Did we forget to be beginners and see what is on the other side?

Try not to use brute force. There is no completion in yoga asanas. Instead, there can be a whole life of exploration. It is often more rejuvenating to breathe and gently advance the stretch than to let your arms and legs just hang and call it a day.

Head-to-Knee Forward Bend (Janu Sirsasana)

Getting In

- Start in Staff Pose (Dandasana), sitting on the floor with your legs straight out in front of you.
- Bend your right knee and draw it in toward your chest with your foot flat on the mat. Grow taller.

- Let your bent knee fall gently toward the floor.
- With your right hand, guide the sole of your right foot to rest on your inner left thigh so your upper thighs create a 90-degree angle.
- Lengthen and balance your spine on the tripod made by your tailbone and sit bones.
- Lengthen your spine over your left leg as you fold your torso forward.
- Either clasp your hands over your left foot, rest your elbows on the floor on either side of your leg, or take hold of your shin or ankle.
- Breathe deeply. Hold for 5 to 10 breaths or longer.
- Release by coming back into Staff Pose.
- Repeat the pose on the other side.

Key Actions

- They call it Head-to-Knee Forward Bend, but that underestimates this pose's potential. If I were going to rename it, I would call it Head-to-Toe Forward Bend, because we focus on extending the torso forward over the long leg, inviting length into the spine while stretching the body from the crown to the toes.
- The foot of your bent leg should remain active and press into the inner thigh of your straight leg, while allowing the inner thigh to press back into the foot to straighten the overall alignment of the pose.
- Your straight leg also remains strong, supporting and grounding the pose. The foot of this leg is flexed.
- In forward bends, try to avoid rounding the back by lengthening the entire spine and allowing the head to move toward the foot.

Modifications

- Beginner: Hold on to a strap wrapped around your outstretched foot to help lengthen your spine. You can also use other props to help you

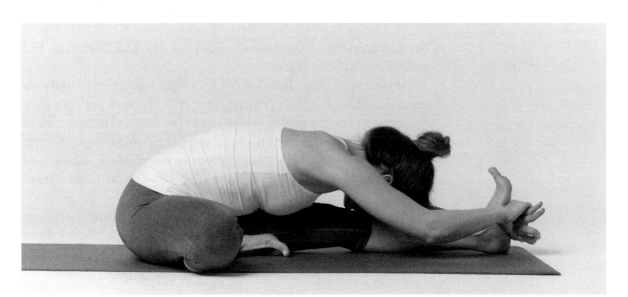

reach your foot and keep your spine long. Consider sitting on a block or a folded blanket. If you experience pain in your bent knee, straighten your leg to relieve the pressure on the knee.

- Intermediate: To deepen the stretch, move your bent knee back even more and press that thigh and knee to the ground.

Benefits

This pose stimulates your internal organs, promotes relaxation, and can help alleviate headaches and high blood pressure.

Contraindications

Do not do this pose if you have knee or lower back issues.

Inspiration

This can be a calming pose, but it is no time to sleep. As you stretch, consider the state you were in when you entered today's practice. Did you feel lazy and lethargic? Hyper and restless? How have you changed? Are you calmer? More energetic? Acknowledge these shifts in your body and mind. Sensations, emotions, thoughts—these are all impermanent things.

Sometimes when students try to reach for their foot, they let their shoulders roll forward too. Give yourself permission to back off and stop letting your shoulders control everything. Gently roll your shoulders away from your ears. The action in your shoulders is a great indicator of how well you are paying attention to your form.

HERON POSE (KROUNCHASANA)

Getting In

- Start in Staff Pose (Dandasana), sitting on the floor with your legs straight out in front of you.
- Bend your right knee. Take hold of your right foot or ankle, and slide your right foot alongside the right hip, with the toes pointing away from you so you are resting on the top of the foot and calf as in Hero Pose (Virasana). Both sit bones and the right calf should be on the mat.
- Bend your left knee. Hold your left foot with both hands, taking your left hand to the outer edge and your right hand to the inner edge of the foot.
- Inhale as you lengthen your spine up through your crown.
- Lift your left leg up and toward you, straightening it as you lift. Press your heel out and flex your toes. Focus on straightening your leg until your foot is above your head.

- Press through your heel to lengthen the stretch.
- Distribute your weight equally on your sit bones. Continue to lengthen your spine. Lift your chest.
- Direct your gaze forward and up toward your left foot.
- Breathe deeply. Hold for 5 to 10 breaths or longer.
- Lower your left foot to the floor.
- To come out, extend both legs in front of you and return to Staff Pose.
- Repeat on the other side.

Key Actions

- This pose builds a tremendous amount of upper body strength. The great quest for many students is extending the upper leg, but this should never be at the expense of collapsing everything else. To avoid collapsing, keep your chest lifted, with your shoulders back and down.
- To stay balanced, focus on the tripod of space between your sit bones and tailbone. Lower your shoulders away from your ears.

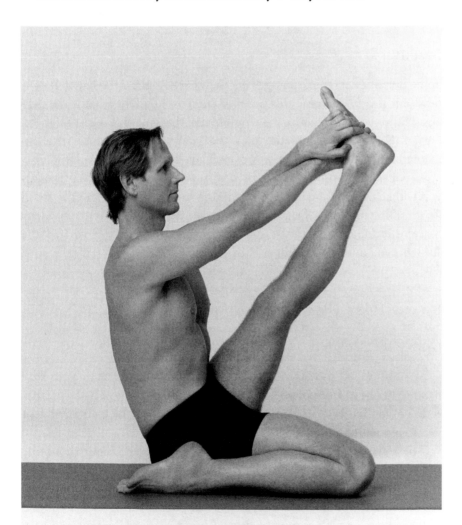

Modifications

- Beginner: If it's difficult to reach your foot, place a strap around the sole of your foot to help keep your chest lifted as you extend your leg.
- Intermediate: You can cross your wrists and take the outside of your left foot with your right hand, and vice versa, for a slightly deeper stretch. If you feel strong and stable, raise your left leg higher. To deepen the stretch, bring your left leg to your torso and rest your forehead on your shin without collapsing your spine. Gaze toward your right foot.
- Advanced: Take the stretch even farther by wrapping your right hand around your left wrist.

Benefits

This elegant pose stretches your hamstrings, hips, and back.

Contraindications

Do not do this pose if you have ankle or knee issues.

Inspiration

Some practitioners think that getting their leg straight is the key to happiness. But if you are doing this pose (or any pose) blindly, what is the purpose? Straightening your leg is a tangible goal that is easy to measure. If you are not also working on quieting the mind, your mood will quickly reveal an incomplete workout. You are only cheating yourself and your community.

As you admire your tall, straight leg, think of the heightened awareness you will achieve by focusing your mind. You now resemble a tall, proud heron. Did you know that the heron is known for its ability to fly high? Start by letting thoughts and distractions gently float away. As you feel the stretch, tune in to your inner silence.

LOTUS POSE (PADMASANA)

Getting In

- Start in Staff Pose (Dandasana), sitting on the floor with your legs straight out in front of you.
- Bend your right knee. With both hands, take hold of your right foot and place it on your left thigh.
- The sole of your foot should be facing up, and its length should be parallel to your left hip crease.
- Lean back onto your sit bones. Bend your left knee. Take hold of your left foot with both hands and place it on your right thigh.
- Place your hands on your knees in Chin Mudra. (Making an O with each index finger and thumb.)

- Straighten and lengthen your spine, find the natural curve in your lumbar spine (lower back), and gently draw in your abdominals.
- Direct your gaze forward.
- Breathe deeply.
- Remain in the pose for as long as you are comfortable.
- Gently come out of the pose by releasing your left foot and then your right; return to Staff Pose.

Key Actions

- The common tendency is to let your feet get sloppy. Keep them active and engaged.
- Use the greatest care as you move your legs and feet into position to avoid any strain on your knees and hips.

Modifications

- Beginner: A great way to know if you are ready for Lotus Pose is to bring one heel at a time close to your navel and turn the top of the foot

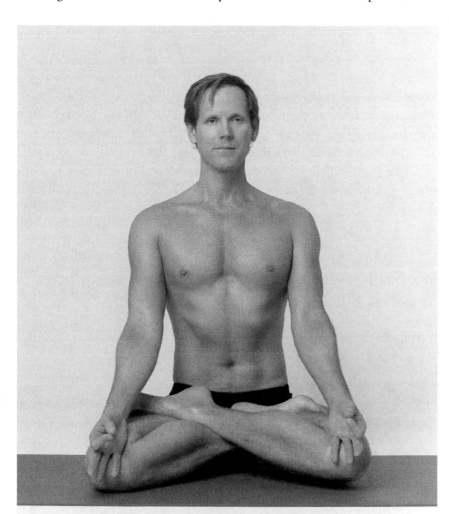

down, making sure your foot stays awake as you place it high up on the opposite thigh. If, on either side, your knee is off the floor, or if one side of your spine is collapsing, you are probably not ready for Lotus Pose. Instead, start with a simple cross-legged sitting position until that is comfortable, or sit in Fire Log Pose (Agnistambhasana). Build up to Half Lotus Pose (Ardha Padmasana), taking only one leg at a time into Lotus Pose, until your flexibility improves. Place your right foot on top of your left thigh and bring your left foot under your right knee. Hold for as long as you are comfortable. Reverse legs and repeat. As with all poses, you can try to yank the fruit off the tree before it is ready, but the fruit won't taste very good.

Benefits

According to ancient texts, this pose destroys all disease and awakens *kundalini*. It also stretches your ankles and knees and calms your nervous system.

Contraindications

Do not do this pose if you have ankle or knee issues.

Inspiration

Lotus Pose is the most famous asana in yoga. As such, students often want to engage in it before their bodies are fully ready. Do not force yourself into this pose. Take the time to do preparatory poses until you are ready. You can still enjoy the physical and mental benefits.

There are well-practiced students who never do Lotus Pose. Any practice should be based on *ahimsa*. There is no essential pose. And no pose should cause pain or harm to your body. You can go the rest of your life without the Lotus Pose and still be happy.

SEATED FORWARD BEND/INTENSE WESTERN STRETCH POSE (PASCHIMOTTANASANA)

Getting In

- Start in Staff Pose (Dandasana), sitting on the floor with your legs straight out in front of you.
- Shift your weight from one side of your buttocks to the other. Adjust your position so your weight is evenly distributed on the tripod created by your sit bones and tailbone.
- Raise your arms straight up to the sky, with palms facing inward and fingers splayed.
- Keeping your core engaged and length in your spine, fold your torso forward, reaching your fingers out toward your toes.

- If you are able, rest your chest on your thighs. Wrap your hands around the soles of your feet.
- Avoid collapsing your spine; rather, lengthen it. If necessary, bend your knees or use a strap around the soles of your feet.
- Stretch it out. With your elbows drawing down, work your shoulders and spine as your shoulders relax away from your ears.
- Engage your thighs, giving your hamstrings the freedom to release safely. Relax your head down, allowing your neck to release any tension.
- Make sure your neck remains comfortable. If gazing forward feels good, do that. If not, consider keeping your neck long and looking down.
- Breathe deeply. Hold for 5 to 10 breaths or longer.
- Come out by rolling back up.

Key Actions

- It is sometimes tempting to drop your head hastily and touch your knees or shins. But I have had my head down, and it has never changed my level of happiness.
- Different schools of thought espouse either flexing your feet or pointing your toes. Whichever of these variations feels best to you is fine, just be sure to keep your legs active and your thighs pressing down. If you are working on keeping your thighs down, keep a slight flex in your feet, with the base of the toes pressing forward but the toes themselves curling back toward you. Find a balance between the flexing and pointing.
- Hinge from your hips. If this means you can keep your legs long, it's all good. If it means you need to bend your knees, that's good too. There are enough variations in this posture that everyone has somewhere to go.

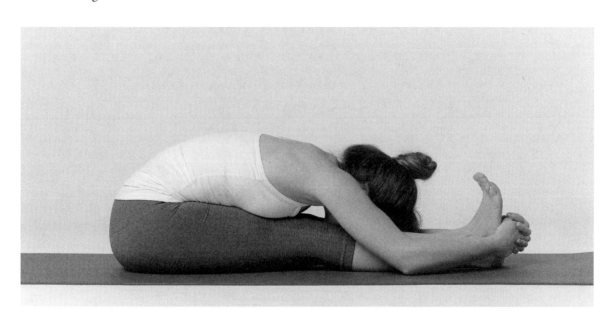

Modifications

- Beginner: If your feet are not accessible, bend your knees or use a strap. You can also hold your ankles or simply rest your hands on your shins.
- Intermediate: If you can easily take hold of your feet, you can lengthen your reach by placing a block at the end of your feet. Reach around the block to further lengthen your torso.

Benefits

This pose gives a rewarding stretch through your hamstrings, groins, and spine that is a tremendous help when you get to other poses such as Shoulderstand, Plow, Pigeon Variations, and Splits.

Contraindications

Do not do this pose if you have knee or lower back issues.

Inspiration

People who are not terribly flexible often come to this pose in one of two ways: either they feel overeager and on a mission to touch their toes, creating a potential for harm from rounding the spine and collapsing the belly; or they don't go anywhere in the pose and instead spend the time looking around the room, comparing themselves to others, and wondering if they will ever be able to rest their chest on their thighs.

It is almost impossible to undo a lifetime of sitting, so don't fret over any tightness revealed in this pose. Be willing to come back and continue to work with great focus on a modification, or simply concentrate on coming back to the breath and count each inhalation and exhalation slowly. When I'm in Seated Forward Bend, I find it helpful to think of a time when I felt truly loved. Then everything seems to open.

WIDE-ANGLE SEATED FORWARD BEND (UPAVISTHA KONASANA)

Getting In

- Start in Staff Pose (Dandasana), sitting on the floor with your legs straight out in front of you.
- Place your hands at your sides.
- Leaning your torso back slightly on your hands, open your legs as wide as you comfortably can. Using your hands for support, slide your buttocks forward slightly and try widening your legs just a little more.
- Make sure your kneecaps are pointing straight up and your feet are flexed.

- Pressing out with your heels, enjoy a good stretch through your hips, thighs, glutes, and shins. Keep your spine straight.
- Bring your hands in front of you and walk them between your legs to fold forward. Make sure you continue to shift your weight back as you fold forward, so that your sit bones remain firmly rooted while keeping both legs fully engaged.
- Assume one of the following arm positions:
  1. Fully extend your arms in front of you with your palms facedown on the mat.
  2. Bend your elbows and place your forearms flat on the floor.
  3. Take hold of the outer edges of your feet, toes, or ankles.

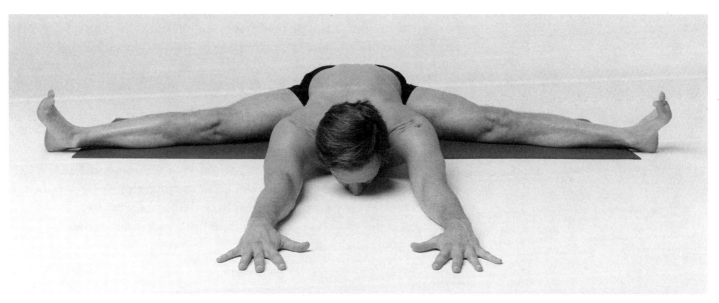

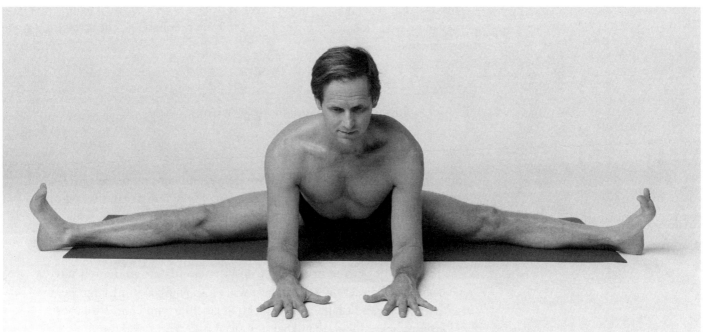

- Draw in your abdominals and feel your spine lengthening up through your neck and crown.
- Direct your gaze forward.
- Breathe deeply. Hold for 5 to 10 breaths or longer.
- To release, walk your hands in and place them behind you for support. Close your legs and return to Staff Pose.

Key Actions

- Your legs are the foundation of the pose. Do not allow your feet to collapse or your legs to turn in.
- Squeeze your quads to give your kneecaps adequate support. Keep your feet flexed so your toes and knees point toward the sky.
- Overstretching can turn this pose into a tug-of-war with your core. Find your comfort level as you stretch your legs and lengthen your spine.

Modifications

- Beginner: If you find that you are rounding forward from your waist instead of folding from your hips, back off. If you feel a painful stretch or pressure behind one or both knees, narrow your legs. Sit on a blanket or a bolster if you need a little extra lift under your hips.
- Intermediate: With your hands curled over the top of your feet, lift your legs off the ground as high as you can with your arms extended, balancing your weight on your sit bones.

Benefits

This deep leg stretch also calms the mind because it is a forward bend. If you can relax in this pose, you can hold it longer, enhancing the stretching benefits.

Contraindications

Do not do this pose if you have lower back issues.

Inspiration

Sometimes we get to a point when we define and confine ourselves (*I'm not flexible and I'll never be able to do this pose*). Then, one day, we let go of these self-imposed limitations. We come back to the beginner's state of honoring the basic principles. Then the pose comes to us, instead of us constantly grasping for the pose.

After years of playing in this pose and thinking I was going nowhere, one day I noticed that my entire chest was on the mat, and my alignment was splendid. In an instant, when I let go of labeling who I am in this pose and limiting myself with that label, I noticed I was comfortable.

Hero Pose (Virasana)

Getting In

- Start in Table Pose (on your hands and knees), with your hips square and your knees aligned under your hips.
- Bring your knees together and position your feet slightly wider than your hips.
- Lower your buttocks to the mat between your heels. Fold your inner calves against your outer thighs with your heels beside your hips.
- Balance your weight on the tripod formed by your sit bones and tailbone.
- Bring your shoulders back and down, and open your chest.
- Rest your hands on top of your thighs or in Chin Mudra (making an O with each index finger and thumb).
- Direct your gaze forward.
- Breathe deeply. Hold for 5 to 10 breaths or longer.
- To come out, place your palms on your heels and lift into a kneeling position.

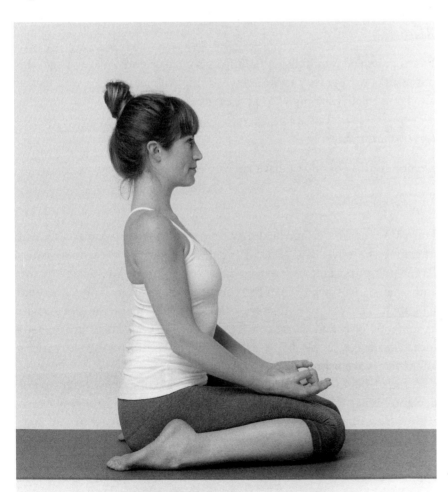

Key Actions

- Keep your hips down without collapsing your lower back.
- Ensure that your knees are protected by keeping your quads active. Energetically, it's as if you are trying to press your thighs into the ground.
- Point your toes straight back and work your baby toes into the floor. Avoid letting your toes splay off to the sides.

Modifications

- Beginner: If the pressure of your ankles against the floor hurts, put a rolled towel under them. Beginning students may want to test their comfort zone. From Table Pose (on your hands and knees), start lowering your buttocks between your feet. As the tension increases across your quads, add a blanket or block beneath your sit bones to relieve the pressure.
- Intermediate: If you feel inspired, clasp your hands together by interlocking your fingers, and press your arms up over your head, with the palms facing the sky. Stretch up through the crown of your head.

Benefits

When practiced mindfully and not from a goal-oriented place of ego, this pose works with gravity to stretch your thighs, knees, ankles, and feet. It also helps to alleviate high blood pressure.

Contraindications

Do not do this pose if you have knee or ankle issues.

Inspiration

Hero Pose can be either healing or very bad for your knees. My rule of thumb is always "If it feels wrong, it *is* wrong." And each day is different. It's important to listen to your body and decide what it wants and what it may need. Do not spend too much time looking at your neighbor. The reality is that we cannot possibly have the same knees as someone else, and if you can avoid replacing your knees, it is a good idea. Your focus should be on exploring your comfort zone and making adjustments accordingly.

A lot of beginner yoga is about getting to know your body as you develop higher levels of flexibility, movement, and conditioning. Inevitably, you will confront a limitation that is not addressed in any yoga book. Never hesitate to discuss any concerns with your yoga teachers who, in the spirit of *seva* (selfless service), are always open to helping you.

Twists

It is often said that twists wring toxins out of the body. It does not matter to me whether or not this claim can be clinically proven. Rather, it is the notion that we open ourselves to the possibility of letting go of toxins—whether physical, mental, or emotional—that is of value. When we squeeze our internal organs, we stimulate their function.

As in other seated poses, it's important to keep a straight spine here. Your oblique abdominal muscles can facilitate a safe twisting of your torso, so it is good to keep your core active during these movements.

Half Lord of the Fishes Pose
(Ardha Matsyendrasana)

Getting In

- Start in Staff Pose (Dandasana), sitting on the floor with your legs straight out in front of you.
- Bend your knees, placing your feet flat on the floor.
- Open your left knee to the left and slide your left foot under your right leg just to the outside of your right hip. Rest your left knee on the mat.
- Lift your right foot (with your hand, if necessary) over your left leg and place the sole on the floor outside your left thigh. Your right knee should be pointing straight up toward the sky.
- Prepare to deepen the twist.
- Place your right hand (fingertips or palm) on the mat behind you.
- Raise your left hand straight up in the air with the palm facing back toward you. Bend your left elbow and place it on the outside of your right knee.
- Turn your head to the right; gaze to the right and then over your right shoulder.
- Breathe deeply. With each inhalation, lengthen your spine. With each exhalation, deepen the twist. Hold for several breaths or longer.
- Gently release to Staff Pose, and repeat on the other side.

Key Actions

- When your hand is placed on the floor behind your back, there is a tendency to lean on it and collapse the length of your spine. Instead, allow that back hand to press into the floor to create a lifting sensation as you twist into the pose. This support helps keep your chest lifted and awakens the breath—and it is safer for your spine.
- Start with the twist in the base of your thoracic (mid) spine. Let your neck turn only as a consequence of the twist.
- Draw in your abdominals for strength and lift.

- To sit taller and breathe easier, find the tripod of space between your tailbone and sit bones, and engage your core for support.
- Keep your bottom leg pressing into the ground.
- Relax your shoulders away from your ears.

Modifications

- Beginner: If it is difficult to keep both sit bones on the floor while you twist, unfold your lower leg and extend it straight out in front of you with the foot flexed. An easier upper arm option is to wrap your upper arm around your knee and hug it toward your body.
- Intermediate: From here, it is possible to move into Bound Half Lord of the Fish Pose (Baddha Ardha Matsyendrasana). The *baddha* (bind) can be harmful if you are pushing the stretch and your muscles beyond your limitations, so move with sensitivity into this more advanced pose. While hugging your right knee with your left arm, bend your left elbow, slide your left arm under your right knee, and reach toward your left hip. Take your right arm behind your back and bring your right hand toward your left hip until you can clasp your hands or fingertips. Draw your shoulder blades in toward your spine to prepare for this deeper twist. Rotate your head to the right, moving your gaze slowly toward the wall in back of you.

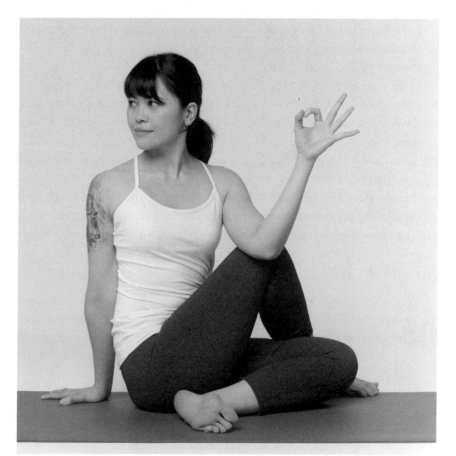

Benefits

This pose energizes your spine; stretches your shoulders, neck, and hips; and can help relieve the symptoms of asthma, backache, menopause, and menstruation.

Contraindications

Do not do this pose if you have back or spine issues.

Inspiration

With every exhalation, I like to allow the breath to move through me as I imagine myself twisting out negative habits and attitudes. Through the inhalation, the twist is an opportunity to think about what you want to bring into your life.

This pose resembles the tail of a fish. According to a Hindu myth, the deity Shiva was on an island explaining the mysteries of yoga to his consort, Parvati. A fish near the shore remained motionless and listened with rapt attention. When Shiva realized that the fish had learned yoga, he blessed it as Matsyendra, Lord of the Fishes. The fish then took a divine form, came on land, and assumed a seated spinal twisting posture that allowed him to fully absorb the teachings. Consider yourself half fish and half human and ever evolving.

I think about how a fish's tail sometimes helps it maneuver into safe and nourishing waters, while on other occasions the tail helps the fish swim away from potential harm. This reminds me to balance energy in a way that brings me into a life-affirming place, where there is no force and no insistence, yet there is the stability to keep me afloat and fully present within the moment.

Some students push the twist into a bind before they are ready, forcing their bodies rather than letting them flow gently, but this often causes the breath to stop moving freely. Listen to your body. If you find that your breath is labored and your spine is collapsing when you're in a bound position, then back off from the bind! The breath must be your guide. If you are choking off your breath to get into a more advanced pose, notice that signal rather than your ego's eagerness to get into the bind. From there, simply choose to back off.

SAGE TWIST (BHARADVAJASANA)

Getting In

- Start in Staff Pose (Dandasana), sitting on the floor with your legs straight out in front of you and your feet flexed.
- Bend your knees and lean onto your left buttock while bringing both knees to the left and your heels to the right.

- Bring your outer left leg and inner right leg to rest on the mat.
- There are two variations of this pose:
  1. Take your right heel outside your right hip and bring the sole of your left foot to rest against the top of your right thigh. Bring your left arm behind your back, placing your left hand or fingertips on the floor behind you. Take your right hand to your left knee.
  2. Bring your left foot into Half Lotus Pose (Ardha Padmasana), placing the top of your left foot on your upper right thigh, toward the hip crease. Turn your torso to the left. Bring your left arm behind your back and slide your fingers into your right hip crease, or take hold of your left foot. Slide your right hand under your left knee, with the palm facing down.
- Rotate your head slowly past your right shoulder, dropping your chin slightly.
- Breathe deeply. Hold for 5 to 10 breaths or longer.
- Release, and repeat on the other side.

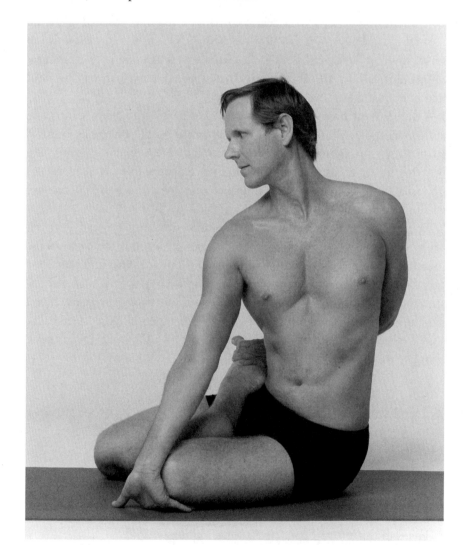

Key Actions

- If you are taking Half Lotus Pose, keep your upper foot active. Feel the top of that foot pressing down on your thigh with your arch awake. Allowing your foot to just hang out is dangerous for your knee and ankle.
- Be sure your spine is straight, stacking each vertebra on top of the next. Avoid focusing the twist on your lower back. Engage your whole spine.
- This is an elegant twist, but it packs a wallop. It is like one-stop shopping: a centering technique with a little bit of Hero Pose (Virasana), a little Lotus Pose (Padmasana), and a great workout for the wrists. Throughout, focus on twisting from your upper back and lengthening your tailbone toward the ground.

Modifications

- Beginner: Place one foot as in Head-to-Knee Forward Bend (Janu Sirsasana) if Half Lotus Pose does not feel comfortable.

Benefits

This pose stretches and strengthens your entire spine, abdominal organs, and kidneys. It also improves digestion.

Contraindications

Do not do this pose if you have high or low blood pressure, or if you are menstruating.

Inspiration

This pose is dedicated to Bharadvaja, one of seven legendary seers. Legend has it he composed the hymns collected in the Vedas. Sage Twist is about elegance, not arrogance. If you have your chin way up, you may feel discomfort in your neck. When taking your gaze back, your chin should be angled down slightly. This adds a certain softness and elegance to the pose.

CHAPTER 16

Restorative Poses

As the name implies, these poses are designed to take you back into a safe place of grounding and calm. There is a softness to them that can bring immense relaxation and clarity of mind. These poses are perfect either on their own after a stressful and chaotic day or at the end of a more vigorous practice. Here you can find deep relaxation whenever you need.

HAPPY BABY POSE (ANANDA BALASANA)

Getting In

- Lie on your back with your feet on the mat and your knees bent skyward.
- Lift your knees toward your torso, bringing your shins parallel to the floor.
- Inhale. Reach for your feet, taking hold of your big toes or your soles from the outer edges. Gently lift your feet until your shins are perpendicular to the floor and your thighs are almost parallel to the floor. Keep your knees bent as you take them wider than torso-width apart, lowering them to the sides of your rib cage. Feel the opening in your groins and hips.
- Lengthen your spine along the mat.
- As the soles of your feet face the sky, root your tailbone down into the ground.
- Direct your gaze up to the ceiling.
- Breathe deeply.
- Rock gently from one side to the other, feeling the stretch in your hips.

- Hold for 5 to 10 breaths or longer.
- To come out, release your legs and reverse out of the pose.

Key Actions

- Happy Baby Pose is typically identified as a restorative pose at the end of class. This is no time to slack off, though. Performing this asana correctly and keeping your entire spine lengthening down the mat requires some effort. One way to deepen the stretch is to engage your core as you focus on flattening your lower back and guiding your tailbone down; otherwise, your hips will want to lift off the floor.
- Do your best to get your shoulders down, and give your biceps a workout. Keep your neck long and relaxed. To counter the lifting of your hips and arching of your lower back, think about your navel moving toward the center of the earth.

Modifications

- Beginner: If taking hold of your feet causes your hips to lift off the ground, take hold of the backs of your thighs or your ankles instead.
- Intermediate: Bring the soles of your feet together and draw them toward your face, allowing your knees to drop open a little more to relieve your hip flexors.

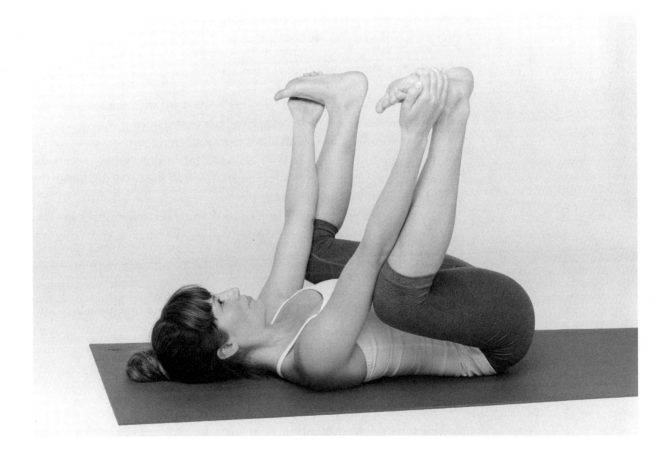

- Advanced: For a deeper stretch, hold your toes as you straighten your legs to the sky. Open your legs wide. Inhale. Exhale and bring your legs back together. Increase the intensity by widening the spread and/or pressing your heels farther out.

Benefits

This only looks like a lazy pose. It is a formidable stretch through your groins, lower back, and hamstrings. It also opens your hips and groins and relieves stress.

Contraindications

Do not do this pose if you have knee or neck issues, or if you are pregnant.

Inspiration

Consider looking at Happy Baby Pose as a really exciting asana and a new beginning rather than as a finishing pose and a time to space out. Truth is, it takes an ample amount of work to get your lower back down and activate your core. Opening your hips and groins will help take some of your other poses to a new level.

RECLINING BOUND ANGLE POSE (SUPTA BADDHA KONASANA)

Getting In

- Start in Bound Angle Pose (Baddha Konasana), with the soles of your feet together and your knees splayed out to the sides.
- Lie on your back by rolling down onto your spine vertebra by vertebra.
- Lift your hips and tuck your tailbone forward so your lower back relaxes toward the floor. Keeping this tuck of the tailbone, lower the hips back down.
- Do not force your knees down. Instead, softly relax your inner groins.
- Extend your arms out to the sides. Or place one hand on your belly and one on your heart.
- Close your eyes.
- Breathe deeply. Hold for 5 to 10 breaths or longer.
- To release, lift onto one elbow, then the other, and finally back up into Bound Angle Pose.

Key Actions

- Continue settling your groins deep into your pelvis.
- Instead of pushing your knees toward the floor in the hope of increasing the stretch, imagine that your knees are floating comfortably on top

of water. As you relax and stay, your groins will naturally begin to drop toward the floor, as will your knees. Invite a softness into your entire pelvic area and upper legs.

- Ensure that your neck is aligned with your spine and your spine is straight.

Modifications

- Beginner: Lay your head on a rolled up towel. If your knees are sore, or if there is too much stretch in your groins, place a prop (block, blanket, or rolled-up towel) under each knee. Whichever method you choose, there should be no strain in your lower back.

Benefits

This pose opens your hips and groins. By encouraging blood flow through your pelvis, it stimulates digestion and your reproductive organs. It also calms the mind.

Contraindications

Do not do this pose if you have knee issues.

Inspiration

Allow your mind to rest with every breath. If you have discomfort, realign the pose until you feel comfortable and relaxed. For all the contorting and bending you do in yoga, remember that the practice is ultimately about stilling the mind and creating a more balanced, harmonious state of being. Once relaxation is achieved in the outer, physical realm, you will begin to find peace in your inner world.

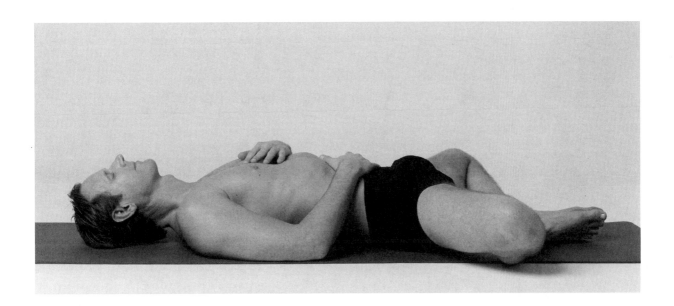

RECLINING HERO POSE (SUPTA VIRASANA)

Getting In

- Start in Hero Pose (Virasana).
- Place your hands behind you. Slowly begin to lower onto your forearms and elbows, then lie on your back, rolling down vertebra by vertebra.
- Extend your arms alongside your body with your palms cupping your heels.
- Direct your gaze up to the sky.
- Breathe deeply. Hold for 5 to 10 breaths or longer.
- Release by moving into Corpse Pose (Savasana).

Key Actions

- Brace your core to protect your lower back as you lower onto the mat. Tuck your tailbone, slide your pelvis forward, and engage the *bandhas*. This will also encourage your spine to lengthen.
- Let your breath and the comfort of your knees and lower back determine how far you go in this pose. Pay great attention to your knees. Splaying them wider than your hips can cause strain. If at any point you feel pain in your knees, hips, or lower back, immediately (but gracefully) lift up out of the pose and find a place that is healing for the painful area.
- While this is a restorative pose, try to keep your legs active by pressing your knees into the ground and guiding them continuously toward each other.

Modifications

- Beginner: If there is stress in your knees or quads, lie back on a blanket, bolster, or other prop to raise your back higher; this will relieve the

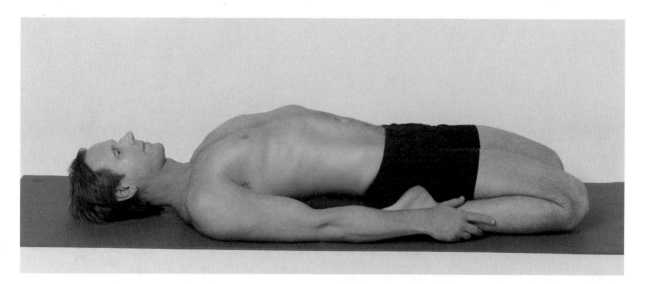

pressure. If the full pose is too difficult, try Reclining Half Hero Pose (Supta Ardha Virasana). Draw your right leg back into Hero Pose and keep your left knee bent with your foot flat on the floor. Then lower carefully onto your back, as you would in the full pose. Come out and repeat on the left side. If you are not ready for this, stay seated in Hero Pose and try modifications with props such as a bolster, folded blankets, or a block. (See the modifications for Hero Pose on page 214.)

Benefits

This pose provides a good stretch of your abdomen, psoas muscles, knees, and ankles.

Contraindications

Do not do this pose if you have back or knee issues.

Inspiration

Only recline when you can find true, honest comfort in Hero Pose. If you cannot sit with your buttocks on the floor between your feet, you should not be reclining. It is not safe for your knees, and you are not ready. Remember, there is no rush, and you can build the pose slowly over time. Focus on developing technique and reward yourself for honoring where you are and investing the time in your physical and mental well-being.

CHAPTER 17

Surya Flow 1

THIS IS A ONE-HOUR SEQUENCE that I designed for early-morning practitioners at our studio. Enjoy!

Minutes 0 to 3

OM
Prayer to teachers:
  Guru Brahma, Guru Vishnu, Guru Devoh Maheswaraha
  Guru Saakshaat Para Brahma, Tasmai Shree Guruve Namaha
Prayer for universal well-being and happiness:
  Lokah Samaastha Sukhino Bhavantu
  OM Shaantih Shaantih Shaantih OM

Minutes 3 to 10

Sun Salutation (Surya Namaskara) A—3 times
Sun Salutation (Surya Namaskara) B—3 times
Big Toe Pose (Padangusthasana)—5 breaths
Hand Under Foot Pose (Padahasthasana)—5 breaths

Minutes 10 to 15

Do each of the following on one side—5 breaths each pose on each side:
  Warrior I Pose (Virabhadrasana I)
  Warrior II Pose (Virabhadrasana II)
  Reverse Warrior Pose (Viparita Virabhadrasana)
  Extended Side-Angle Pose (Utthita Parsvakonasana)

On the same side, flow through each of the following—5 breaths each
for the standing poses:
Warrior II Pose
Reverse Warrior Pose
Warrior II Pose
Flow to the other side via exhaling to Four-Limbed Staff Pose, inhaling to Upward-Facing Dog Pose, and exhaling to Downward-Facing Dog Pose.
Flow to the other side and repeat the sequence.
Return to the first side, and flow to Warrior I Pose. From here, turn your back heel up so you're on the ball of the back foot in Lunge Pose, bring your hands to prayer position (Anjali Mudra) at your heart, twist into Revolved Side-Angle Pose (Parivritta Parsvakonasana), and hold for 5 breaths.
Flow to the other side via exhaling to Four-Limbed Staff Pose, inhaling to Upward-Facing Dog Pose, and exhaling to Downward-Facing Dog Pose.

Minutes 15 to 20

Do each of the following to one side—5 breaths each:
Warrior I Pose
Warrior II Pose
Extended Triangle Pose (Utthita Trikonsasana)
Half-Moon Pose (Ardha Chandrasana)
Revolved Half-Moon Pose (Parivritta Ardha Chandrasana)
Bring both hands down and step back into Warrior I Pose.
Bring your hands into prayer position at your heart then open into Warrior II Pose.
Flow to the other side via Four-Limbed Staff Pose, Upward-Facing Dog Pose, and Downward-Facing Dog Pose, and repeat the sequence. (These are on an exhale-inhale-exhale.)

Minutes 20 to 25

Mountain Pose (Tadasana)—3 to 5 breaths
Standing balance options—5 breaths each pose on each side:
Tree Pose (Vrksasana)
Extended Hand to Big Toe Pose (Utthita Hasta Padangusthasana)
Lord of the Dance Pose (Natarajasana)
Chair Pose (Utkatasana)—5 breaths
Crow/Crane Pose (Bakasana)—5 breaths
Carefully jump or step back into Four-Limbed Staff Pose, inhale to Upward-Facing Dog, and exhale to Downward Dog, where you then hold for 5 breaths.

Minutes 25 to 30

Inhale as you assume Plank Pose (Phalakasana); hold for 5 breaths.
Slowly lower to the floor for back strengthening:
  Locust Pose (Salabhasana) variation 1, with arms alongside your
    body (5 breaths)
  Relax for a few seconds with your head turned to one side, big toes
    touching, and heels apart.
  Locust Pose variation 2, with arms out in front, arms out to the
    sides at shoulder level, or hands behind the back with fingers
    laced—5 breaths
  Relax for a few seconds with your head turned to the other side,
    big toes touching, and heels apart.
  Bow Pose (Dhanurasana)—5 breaths

Minutes 30 to 40

  Push up to Plank Pose.
  Do 5 push-ups.
  Downward-Facing Dog Pose—5 breaths
  Child's Pose (Balasana)—5 breaths
  Raise up on your hands and knees; walk your knees forward into Hero
    Pose (Virasana) or Reclining Hero Pose (Supta Virasana); hold for
    10 breaths.
  Move from Hero Pose to sit on your heels. Then sit to the left of your
    heels and place your right foot on the floor outside your left thigh
    to go into Half Lord of the Fishes Pose (Ardha Matsyendrasana);
    hold for 5 breaths on each side.
  Seated Forward Bend (Paschimottanasana)—10 breaths
  Head-to-Knee Forward Bend (Janu Sirsasana)—5 breaths on each side
  Bound Angle Pose (Baddha Konasana)—5 breaths
  Release, then lower slowly onto your back with your knees to your chest.

Minutes 40 to 45

  Core Work: (Do any combination of these exercises for a total of 5 or
    more minutes.)
    Single and double Leg Lifts
    Bicycle
    Revolved Abdomen Pose (Jathara Parivartasana)

Minutes 45 to 47

  Do two backbends for 5 breaths each:
    Bridge Pose
    Upward Bow Pose (Urdhva Dhanurasana)

Minutes 47 to 49

> Reclining Bound Angle Pose (Supta Baddha Konasana)—5 breaths
> Reclining Twist (bring your knees to your chest then take your knees
> over to each side)—5 breaths on each side

Minute 49 to 51

> Happy Baby Pose (Ananda Balasana)—5 breaths

Minutes 51 to 53

> Seated meditation—2 minutes

Minutes 53 to 58

> Corpse Pose (Savasana)—5 minutes

Minutes 58 to 60

> Closing chant and blessing—2 minutes

CHAPTER 18

Special Considerations

Each student of yoga is unique and may come to the practice with special considerations. It's important to know what your own general health is like and any particulars that could affect (or be affected by) this practice or any new form of exercise.

Although this book does not attempt to address the vast science of therapeutic yoga, there still are some basic guidelines for more common concerns like high blood pressure and pregnancy.

Blood Pressure Issues

Yoga can be highly beneficial for both high and low blood pressure. As a general guideline, here is what you should know, but as with any new movement practice, be sure to check with your physician before beginning.

If you have high blood pressure, the poses that are most beneficial are seated and supine poses, including many forward bends. Restorative poses are especially helpful, so allow yourself to luxuriate in these.

Avoid poses that place your head below your heart or in which you feel any pressure in your throat or temples. In poses that call for your arms to be held over your head, bring your hands to your hips or to prayer position (Anjali Mudra) instead. Also avoid poses that compress the front of your diaphragm, such as some backbends. If your blood pressure is regulated with medication, it is likely safe for you to practice many of the poses, but be sure to check with your physician.

If you have low blood pressure, the poses that are most beneficial are backbends and twists, both of which stimulate the kidneys, and certain inversions, which bring pressure to your head. However, practice inversions with caution. Work with a qualified teacher to learn what modifications are best for you.

Avoid poses that require you to stand up quickly. To modify these, simply release the poses slowly and mindfully.

Bhakti Flow Yoga is a lovely practice no matter what your blood pressure is. Inhale as you rise up or release poses, and take your time! If you ever feel dizzy or light-headed, bring your head below your heart or simply sit or lie down.

Pregnancy

If you are expecting, please consult with your health care provider before beginning any new exercise program. It's important that you do not get overheated. If you feel too warm, drink water, breathe through your mouth, or pause in a restorative pose until you cool down.

There are several guidelines for pregnant students practicing *vinyasa* (flow-based) yoga. Here are a few tips to help you safely and fully enjoy your practice:

- Pregnancy causes the body to release a hormone called relaxin that, true to its name, relaxes the ligaments so much that pregnant women often overstretch during yoga without realizing they are doing so. To avoid this, back off a bit from the stretching, and instead focus on the breathing and strengthening aspects of your practice.
- Deep twists that originate in the belly are not healthy for pregnant women, because they can put undue pressure on the uterus. Instead, twist lightly from your shoulders. Your shoulders and chest can open a bit, but your abdomen should not rotate.
- The type of jumps we sometimes do during the *vinyasa* practice can present a very slight risk of dislodging the fertilized egg during the early stages of pregnancy. So step or walk through your *vinyasa* transitions. (And it won't be comfortable to jump later on as well.)
- Instead of practicing any type of *pranayama* that requires breath retention or rapid breathing, such as Kapalabhati (Cleansing Breath), you can practice your "birthing" breath. Ask a teacher to demonstrate, if you're not sure how to do it.
- You should not practice inversions, since you run the risk of tipping over or falling ungracefully to the floor. Legs-Up-the-Wall Pose (Viparita Karani) where you simply lie on your back with your legs up a wall, perhaps with a blanket under the sacrum or head, is a gentle variation with benefits similar to full inversions.
- Avoid deep backbends such as Wheel Pose (Urdhva Dhanurasana). A supported variation of Bridge Pose (Setu Bandha Sarvangasana) is a nice modification.
- During pregnancy, the abdominal muscles naturally relax to accommodate your growing belly. Abdominal poses that tighten this area, such as Full Boat Pose (Paripurna Navasana), are contraindicated.
- Belly squishers such as Cobra Pose (Bhujangasana) are also no-no's.

You can practice them through your first trimester, but avoid them later in your pregnancy.

• As your pregnancy progresses, your doctor may advise you to avoid lying on your back for long periods of time. At this point (or at any point when it feels natural), you can practice Corpse Pose (Savasana) on your side.

I could go on and on about how great yoga is for pregnant women and how important it is to practice mindfully and with full body awareness, but these guidelines should provide a good start.

Thank You

Thank you for joining me on this journey.

May your day be filled with softness and ease and at least some element of surprise—just enough to keep you thoroughly entertained and appreciative of life's brevity, beauty, fragility, and many kindnesses. Just remember to take a few nice long breaths and, with each exhalation, smile at the wonder that is your life and all that has been entrusted to you. How blessed we are!

Acknowledgments

Thank you!

Lori Snyder, my "editor extraordinaire" and the best cheerleader I've ever known. She has been a beacon of light on this journey. I could not have done this without her. Working with Lori over the past couple of years has been one of the best experiences of my life. Thank you, dear Lori!

My literary agent, Kathleen Rushall, of Marsal Lyon Literary Agency. Thank you for taking a chance on me.

Beth Frankl, editor for Shambhala Publications / Trumpeter Books. Thank you for believing in me and helping me make this a reality.

Ben Gleason, assistant editor for Shambhala Publications / Trumpeter Books. Thank you for helping bring clarity and accuracy to each sentence.

Photographer: The incomparable Thayer Allison Gowdy and her amazing agent, Rachel Olmstead.

My co-models: Adam LaPierre, Andrea Smith, and Ann Santos.

Research assistants: Matthew D. Milligan, Reena Ghosh, and Dr. Anna Kaplan.

Proofreader pals: Adam La Pierre, Sherry Farr, Allen Black, Jennifer Jarrett, Joslyn Hamilton, and Allyn Hall.

Joshua Greene, the sweetest man and most patient assistant on earth. Thank you for your many roles and for always flowing in just the right direction. Thank you for saying yes, especially those times you didn't mean to!

Andrea Smith, thank you for your many years of support and keeping me organized and always down to earth. Your faithful service and friendship have fueled me in the very best of ways.

Thank you to these very special supporters: Laurene Powell-Jobs, Stacey Rubin, Linda Hothem, Matthew Monahan, Judith Hellman, and Karin Bauer, who all showed up at just the right time. You have made many dreams come true. Thank you for going above and beyond. Thank you for taking a chance.

To Wah!, my dear friend, who blends music and love to the point that there is no longer any distinction. Thank God we found each other.

To all the Bhakti Flow teachers and assistants who have listened to me repeat the same stories and jokes over and over again and have been kind enough to remind me which foot goes forward when I just can't seem to remember.

A special thank you to Andrea Maltzer, Sherry Farr, and Jennifer Jarrett for never blinking. They have stuck by my side through thick and thin with just the right infusion of respect, fun, and humor. I couldn't ask for better company.

To Ahmed Shalabi, for his beautiful heart, unwavering friendship, and for never letting go of the music from the 1980s.

To Vivi Letsou and Eraj Shakib, who, many years ago, introduced me to my second home of Greece and allowed me to introduce Bhakti Flow to the beautiful yoga community there.

Thank you to my trailblazer yogi friends who keep this path clean, clear, and evolving: Baron Baptiste, Bryan Kest, Luke Ketterhagen, Jai Uttal, Steph Snyder, and Jason Crandell. And a special thank-you to the truly missed Georg Feuerstein and to his dear wife, Brenda. Your gifts are forever ingrained in all of us.

I bow to my dearest teacher, Panditji Rajmani Tigunait. May my efforts do justice to the kindnesses you have bestowed upon me.

To my eight beautiful brothers and sisters, Michael, Patti, Jeannie, Mark, Peggy, Lori, Patrick, and Mallory. I love you all so very much.

And most of all, I dedicate this work—and my humble life—to my dearest love, Kevin, who practices the most authentic yoga without ever touching a mat. May my life touch your life always for the better, just as yours has always done for mine.

It is an honor and a privilege having each one of you in my life.

Index of Poses